SUPERFIT

SUPERFIT

Royce Gracie's Ultimate Martial Arts Fitness and Nutrition Guide

Royce Gracie and James Strom

with Kid Peligro

INVISIBLE CITIES PRESS
MONTPELIER, VERMONT

Invisible Cities Press
50 State Street
Montpelier, VT 05602
www.invisiblecitiespress.com

Photographs by Tom Page, TomPagePhotography.com

Library of Congress Cataloging-in-Publication Data

Gracie, Royce.
Superfit : Royce Gracie's ultimate martial arts fitness and nutrition guide /
Royce Gracie and James Strom with Kid Peligro.
p.   cm.
ISBN 1-931229-33-3
1. Martial arts—Training. 2. Martial artists—Nutrition.
3. Physical fitness. I. Title: Royce Gracie's ultimate martial arts fitness.
II. Strom, James. III. Peligro, Kid. IV. Title.
GV1102.7.T7G73 2004
613.7'148—dc22

2003021163

Royce Gracie wishes to thank Century Martial Arts, Mike Swain,
Gold's Gym, Oakley, and Atama Kimonos for their support.

Anyone practicing the techniques in this book does so at his or her own risk. The authors and the publisher assume no responsibility for the use or misuse of information contained in this book or for any injuries that may occur as a result of practicing the techniques contained herein. The illustrations and text are for informational purposes only. It is imperative to practice these holds and techniques under the strict supervision of a qualified instructor. Additionally, one should consult a physician before embarking on any demanding physical activity.

Printed in The United States of America

Book design by Peter Holm, Sterling Hill Productions

CONTENTS

Introduction

Welcome to *Superfit,* the most advanced fitness program for martial artists ever developed. If you are a serious martial artist, you have undoubtedly used other fitness books or workout routines in the past, and you've probably been frustrated by them. The martial arts demand a unique blend of power, quickness, agility, flexibility, and endurance from their practitioners, and most fitness programs just aren't designed to deliver this. They may make you an iron-pumping hulk who can't move on his feet, or a top runner who couldn't punch his way through a paper bag, or even a strong, fast football player who has no flexibility. What they won't make you into is a top martial artist.

James and Royce have been working together for years to develop the program you want, and in your hands you hold the perfected version of it. We know it works, because Royce has used it for years in competition and has consistently beaten larger opponents with it. Its three-pronged system combines stretching, exercises, and nutrition to hone you into a fighting machine.

Stretching is often underrated, but it is as essential to proper fitness as exercise and nutrition. Because it is responsible for increased flexibility, it is a key component in the martial artist's toolkit. It makes sure that your body is ready for training each day, thus decreasing the chance of injury. Too often, unprepared fighters actually hurt themselves with training because they haven't prepped their bodies.

The exercises presented here are designed to work every part of your fighting arsenal. They will not only increase your strength, endurance, and agility, they will also train your neurons to react instantly to situations of all kinds.

Good nutrition is essential for two reasons: it builds the strong bones and muscles necessary for fighting, and it can ensure that you have a ready supply of fuel on the day of competition. *Superfit* combines the best of modern and ancient nutritional sciences to give you a meal plan that takes the high-nutrient diet today's athletes need and works it into Royce's family diet, a famous system of food combining developed by Royce's family over decades and proven to be one of the secrets of their remarkable success.

It is important to remember that stretching, exercise, and nutrition are not separate components that stand alone; they are interconnected. For instance, if you want to have power at certain angles, you have to become flexible enough to achieve those angles comfortably. Take the example of a competitor who has tight hamstrings. These pull the hips back and rotate them, preventing him from getting much height on a front kick. He will also have little power as he kicks higher, and he will be unable to defend the guard very well, as he can't stand to have his legs pushed over his head. Moreover, even if he has stretched and has loose hamstrings, if he hasn't eaten enough protein while training, he won't have the muscles to deliver any power with a front kick, and if he hasn't eaten sufficient carbohydrates the day of competition, he won't have the energy in his muscles to make them work at their peak.

The point is that to be fit and functional you have to eat right, exercise properly, and stretch regularly. Once you commit yourself to these three objectives, you will notice such a change in your lifestyle and how you feel about yourself that you will become addicted to the good feeling and never go back.

Meet the Authors

Royce Gracie

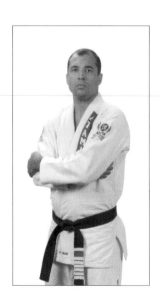

Royce Gracie shocked the world when he entered the Ultimate Fighting Championship (the largest pay-per-view event at that time) in 1993 as an unknown and defeated much larger opponents in record time. He went on to win two more UFCs and other events. In doing so, he introduced America to Brazilian jiu-jitsu, now the most in-demand martial art in the world. Royce's stamina is legendary. The result of natural ability and his unique training program, it has allowed him to achieve superhuman feats, including being the first person in no-holds-barred fighting history to defeat four opponents in a single night, and fighting the longest match in modern no-holds-barred history—a 90-minute marathon at the Tokyo Dome in 2000 in front of 50,000 spectators. Royce trains top-level martial artists, teaches international seminars, and continues to fight professionally.

James Strom

James Strom began his strength coaching with the Los Angeles Rams in the 1980s, where he worked with Eric Dickerson, Jim Everett, and many other stars. From 1993 to 1998 he was head strength coach for the University of Southern California Trojans, where he was in charge of all nineteen varsity sports, both male and female. Some of the many athletes he worked with were basketball player Lisa Leslie, swimmer Janet Evans, and football players Willie McGinest, Keyshawn Johnson, Tony Boseli, and Jason Sehorn. In 1998 James became an exclusive private trainer. His clients have included football players Andre Rison and Keyshawn Johnson, actor Forrest Whitaker, and Royce Gracie. James and Royce met in 1995 after James wrote an article about volleyball strength and conditioning for *Muscle and Fitness* magazine. James lives and teaches in Los Angeles.

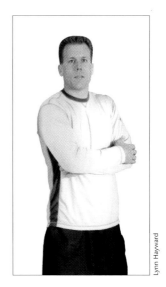

Kid Peligro

One of the leading martial arts writers in the world, Kid Peligro is responsible for regular columns in *Grappling* and *Gracie Magazine*, as well as the most widely read Internet MMA news page, *ADCC News*. He has been the author or coauthor of an unprecedented string of bestsellers in recent years, including *The Gracie Way, Brazilian Jiu-Jitsu Theory and Technique, Brazilian Jiu-Jitsu Self-Defense Techniques, Brazilian Jiu-Jitsu Black Belt Techniques,* and *Brazilian Jiu-Jitsu Submission Grappling Techniques.* A black belt in jiu-jitsu, Kid's broad involvement in the martial arts has led him to travel to the four corners of the Earth as an ambassador for the sport that changed his life. He makes his home in San Diego.

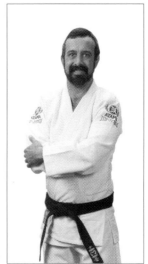

How to Use This Book

This book is intended for a variety of people, from advanced martial artists to perfect beginners. To get the most out of this book, the first thing you must do is evaluate your physical condition. Are you a total beginner? Haven't lifted a finger in years? Place yourself in group A. If you are an intermediate practitioner who regularly exercises but doesn't have a specific program, put yourself in group B. If you are an advanced practitioner, in good shape and just looking for new ideas to add to your workouts, consider yourself group C!

If you are in category C (an advanced practitioner), you will scan the book, look closely at some exercises in part 2 that you haven't seen before, and add them to your routine. You may also want to try Royce's advanced workout routine for a period of six weeks, noting the benefits you get from it, then tweaking it by adding some of your own favorite exercises. But remember, this is Royce's method to increase stamina, strength, and fitness for martial artists. Typically, if you are an advanced practitioner, you have done your research and have a great deal of knowledge in training and conditioning already. You should look to pick up four to six new exercises or one or two new concepts that will turbocharge your workouts and take you to the next level.

If you are in group B (an intermediate practitioner who doesn't have a regular or specific exercise program), this book will greatly benefit you. We recommend that you first look over the exercises in part 2 and familiarize yourself with them and their nomenclature. Next, read the entire introduction and get to know what the *Superfit* system is all about. Then begin the intermediate workouts in part 3 and do them for four consecutive weeks. After that, if you feel you have what it takes, proceed to the advanced workouts for six more weeks. These workouts not only give you an expert pattern to follow, but they will also condition your body and mind to a regular exercise program.

If you are just beginning to exercise, the first thing you need to do after reading the introduction is to go directly to the beginner's workout section in part 3. Next, consult parts 1 and 2 to learn the proper way to perform each required stretch and exercise as it arises in the workout. It is important to note that there will be a trial-and-error period in which you learn to select the proper weights for each exercise. Make sure you note those start weights; you may even consider copying the workout pages and making notes on them. The key to proper selection is to use enough weight that you have difficulty executing the last rep. If you can't do the required number of repetitions, you are using too much weight. If you get to the last rep and you still can do many more, you are using too little weight.

After you have learned to execute each exercise correctly and determined your correct start weights, it is time to start the workouts. Make sure you don't overdo it, especially if you haven't exercised in some time. As noted, you will see a lot of gain in the early stages (not instantaneously, of course) and in three to five weeks you should be developing muscle strength, agility, and new energy.

If you are not sure which category you fit into, start with the beginner's workout. If, at the end of the workout, you do not feel tired or that you made any effort, then go to the intermediate, and so forth. Likewise, if you believe you are intermediate level and find that you cannot handle the intermediate workout, step back and use the beginner's program. Be honest with yourself. *Superfit* is a system designed to get you in as good a shape as you need to be, whether you are a couch potato who wants to get more active, an athlete who wants to step up his game, or a serious martial artist who wants to reach the top level. The key, however, is not to get ahead of yourself and end up either injuring yourself or giving up midway because the workouts are too tough for your current conditioning. Remember that it is not important where you start but where you end up! At the end of the program you should have gained significant benefits in fitness.

We recommend that groups A and B work out for four weeks, then take a two-week active rest period. Group C should work out for six weeks, then take the same two-week active rest. Only after the active rest phase should you proceed to the next level. In some cases, this will mean actually moving from one workout to another; in others, it will mean returning to the workout that you have just finished, but changing the sequence of exercises or stepping up the difficulty of your daily routines. Note that the advanced workout routine described in part 3 is not six weeks long. At the end of it, you will go to the intermediate routine, add an exercise to each daily routine, and continue until you have worked out for six weeks.

You may also notice that many of the exercises in part 2 are not referred to in the workouts. These exercises are presented as options because it is important to modify your workouts as you progress to keep yourself from plateauing or getting bored. When you are ready for a new challenge, you will find that you can easily replace scheduled exercises with the "extra" exercises in part 2 for maximum benefit.

Because stretching is an extremely important part of exercising and total fitness, part 1 of this book is devoted to it. If you are flexible, not only will you be able to perform better in life and in sports, but you will also greatly reduce your injuries as your muscles and joints will have a greater effective range of motion. Begin slowly as you work through part 1, mastering each of the stretches and learning the proper sequence of them so that you can go from one to the next in the routine without having to consult the book. It may sound simplistic, but stretching takes time, effort, and determination. The more you stretch, the better you will be at it and the greater your gains and rewards. Contrary to your progress with the exercises (where you will make your largest gains in the initial phase), stretching is most difficult in the beginning and even the smallest gains are not made without great effort. But as you get settled into a regular stretch routine and learn to relax and breathe, your muscles and joints will release and you will have very rewarding results. Remember, stretching is about relaxation, so when you are ready to start your stretching routine, make sure you allow your body and mind to do just that: relax!

Similar to stretching, a good diet will not give you immediate results, but after some time you will notice greater vitality and more energy. The diet we present in part 4, Royce's family diet, is all about correct food combinations. When followed properly, the diet enhances digestion by allowing your body to absorb nutrients without having to struggle to process food. There is nothing worse than heartburn or an upset stomach after a meal; these are indicators that your body is not concentrating on acquiring the nutrients from the meal but rather fighting to digest it. Especially if you are in a serious exercise program, this struggle will slow down your gains, greatly affect your ability to recuperate from the workouts, and hinder your healing processes. As with other parts of the *Superfit* system, begin the diet slowly. Understand its principles first, and then begin to develop meals that fit the diet and use them in lieu of your regular meals. Little by little, you can begin to incorporate other food combinations, and little by little you will not only easily change your eating habits but be on your way to feeling better and more energetic!

— PART ONE —

Warming Up and Stretching

Being flexible enhances anyone's life, but for martial artists it can mean the difference between victory and defeat. Their bodies are their instruments, and the ability to perform efficiently at their peak without injuries is paramount to a successful career. A flexible person is not only less prone to injury, due to greater range of motion in muscles and joints, but also is able to deliver power more efficiently at a greater variety of angles and positions.

Additionally, with flexibility comes the ability to be comfortable and effective in situations where a less flexible person would struggle. There are three types of flexibility: static, functional, and ballistic. Static flexibility is the ability to get the most out of your range of motion in a slow, steady stretch. Functional flexibility involves stretching in one continuous motion while performing a task, such as raising your leg to mimic a high kick or defend the guard pass. Ballistic flexibility involves one's ability to reach the apex of the stretch in a ballistic—or explosive—situation, such as delivering a high kick, performing a throw, or pitching a baseball. The stretches demonstrated in this book were developed specifically to meet the needs of martial artists, who must not only have excellent range of motion at rest but also be able to put that flexibility to work in functional and ballistic circumstances.

Just as flexibility varies from individual to individual, it also varies from joint to joint and side to side within an individual. A person may have very flexible hamstrings, for example, but be very stiff in the hips. No matter how flexible you are, significant improvement can be achieved with regular warm-ups and stretching exercises, such as the ones Royce demonstrates here.

Warming Up

It is extremely important to warm up your joints and muscles prior to stretching or working out! Without proper warm-up, any attempt to stretch the "cold" joints and muscles may lead to injuries. Much as you let your car warm up before leaving your garage to make certain the oil has reached every bearing and valve in the engine, proper warm-up will "lubricate" your joints and muscle fibers with fresh blood and oxygen, assuring their best performance.

Pre-stretch warm-ups should consist of circling your hips, knees, and ankles while standing, followed by rotating each arm, circling your neck, and moving your head from side to side. Ideally, you should do a pre-stretch warm-up routine, then proceed to the Gracie Stretch Routine (GSR for short) described below, followed by your workout and a second GSR. This is especially important if you are preparing for a specific event such as a competition or a fight. The completeness of this program will not only give you power and explosion benefits but will also increase your ability to perform in a wide range of angles and motions. On those days when your time is really limited, you still need to squeeze the workout into your schedule if you want to progress. In this circumstance, you might consider dropping the stretch routines, but don't drop the warm-up! It is essential for keeping you from injury.

Stretching

The Gracie Stretch Routine has been used and refined by Royce for years. It is a complete martial arts stretch routine that, when mastered, will render you more powerful, flexible, and less prone to injury. We recommend that you do the complete GSR at least four times a week. However, as noted above, we know that sometimes this is not feasible, especially on the days you are going to do the Superfit workouts. For those days when you know that you really won't have the necessary amount of time to complete the warm-ups, the regular 40-stretch GSR, and the workout, Royce has devised the Abbreviated Gracie Stretch Routine (AGR). This shortened version will still give you the benefits of stretching the most important parts of the body, but in a shorter amount of time. It consists of stretches 1, 2, 3, 4, 6, 10, 12, 14, 16, 18, 21, 22, 23, 24, 27, 28, 30, 31, 32, and 35. Those stretches are marked "AGR" in the stretch routine below.

For all stretches it is important to relax and breathe properly. The general rule of thumb is to exhale into your stretch. Do not bounce back and forth into any stretch except as noted, and do not push yourself beyond your limits! If you feel muscle or tendon pain when you are stretching, your body is telling you that you have reached your limit.

Stop right there or even ease up a little, try to relax and breathe, and stay at that position for 30 seconds while you breathe and visualize that body part stretching. While you will reach "sticking" points in any stretch, your ability to breathe and to concentrate on relaxing the tight area will lead to steady progress.

One of the secrets of the GSR is that most of the stretches have beginner and advanced variations. If you haven't stretched in a while or are not sure how flexible you are, start with the beginner's options and progress to the advanced slowly. You can accelerate your progress by stretching every day and by adjusting some of your daily movements to reflect the stretch routine. For example, if you have to pick something up from the ground, bend at the waist and stretch your hamstrings rather than bending at the knees and lowering your body. If you work a desk job, try placing one leg on the desk to stretch it while you talk on the phone, or try doing shoulder and neck stretches throughout the day. When you can do the beginner stretches easily, try the advanced. But always listen to your body before you commit to doing the advanced variations. Better to spend a little more time at the beginner level than risk injury by advancing too quickly. By following these principles you will improve your stretching naturally and seamlessly.

For competitors who have mastered the regular stretch routine and are looking for extreme results—like preparing for an important match or a professional fight—we have included an advanced routine of two-person stretches. Because they involve a partner, they are a little more difficult and less convenient to perform. Start slowly and make sure to communicate with your partner when you are reaching your limit or "sticking" points. It is important to stop, breath, and relax at those points; after that, you may be able to continue stretching even further, blowing past your limits. If performed regularly and properly, the advanced stretches will take you to a new level of competition.

Both stretch routines below are presented in the same order that Royce performs them. He believes these to be the ideal sequence for himself and other martial artists, as you proceed from stretch to stretch and cover most of the muscles and joints involved in practicing martial arts. Where the stretch only shows one side, make sure that you stretch to both sides.

GRACIE STRETCH ROUTINE GSR

One-Person Stretch Routine

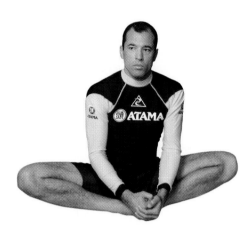

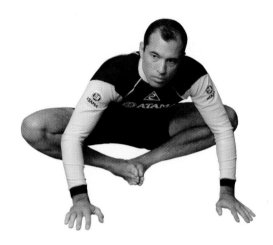

AGR **1.** Sit on the floor with your back straight and your heels touching each other. Hold your feet or your ankles and try to bring your knees to the ground. You may help the stretch by pressing down on your thighs with your elbows. **Advanced:** Lean forward with your torso and try to put your face on the ground.

AGR **2.** Continuing the stretch, slide your feet away from your body slightly, place both hands on the ground in front of you, and lower your torso forward to the ground. Exhale as you move forward.

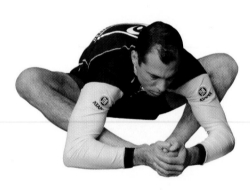

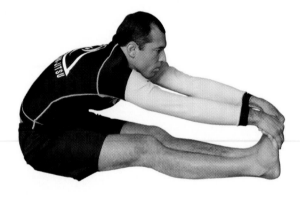

AGR **3.** Extend your feet farther forward and do the same. Try to place your chest on the ground.

AGR **4.** Sit on the floor with your legs extended in front of you. Keep your knees as straight as possible. Lower your torso forward and try to grab your feet with your hands. If you can't reach that far, bend your knees slightly or grab your ankles instead. Again exhale as you stretch forward. **Advanced:** Pull your toes toward you for extra stretch.

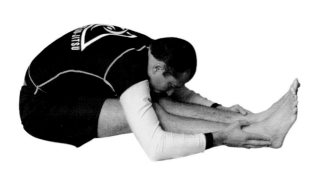

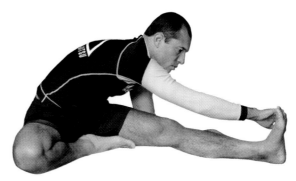

5. Advanced: Lower your torso completely until it touches your thighs.

AGR **6.** Sit on the floor, left leg straight and the other bent with the foot touching the opposite thigh. Keep your back straight a much as possible and lean forward. Try to touch your toes with your right hand. **Advanced:** Grab the outside of your foot with your right hand, thumb facing down.

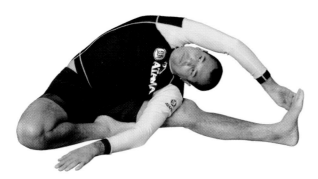

7. Slide your left arm across and reach over with your right arm as you try to grab your foot. **Advanced:** Reach out with your left hand, forcing your torso to twist.

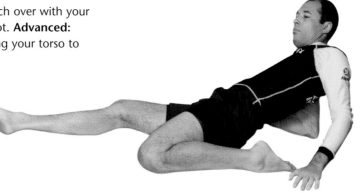

8. With your right leg straight forward and left leg curled back, lean back slowly. You should feel the stretch in your left quadriceps (the top of the thigh).

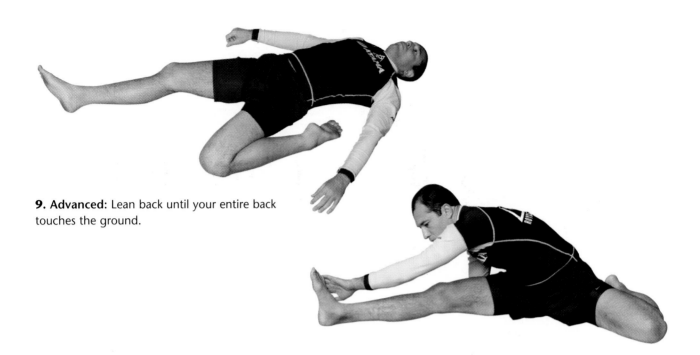

9. Advanced: Lean back until your entire back touches the ground.

AGR **10.** Keeping your right leg forward and left leg tucked, lean forward with your back straight and grab your toes with your left hand. **Beginner:** Start out leaning forward and grabbing your ankle with your right hand to help the stretch. **Advanced:** Grab the outside of your foot with your left palm, thumb down, and pull your foot to you.

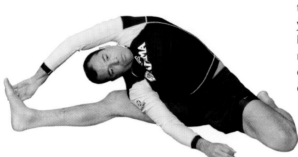

11. Shoot your right arm across and reach over with your left arm to grab your toes. **Beginner:** Reach over your head and lean forward as you exhale.

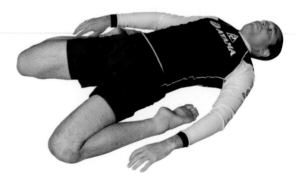

AGR **12.** Kneel down on the floor. Have your feet slightly separated so you can have your buttocks touching the floor. Begin to lean back. **Beginner:** Control your descent with your palms on the ground. **Advanced:** Continue until your entire back touches the ground.

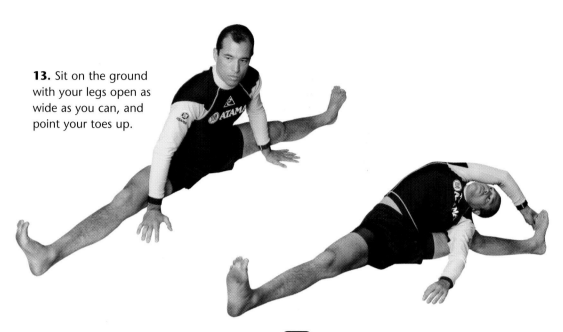

13. Sit on the ground with your legs open as wide as you can, and point your toes up.

AGR **14.** Reach over your head with your arms and try to grab your opposite foot. Reach in with your opposite arm to help out the stretch. **Beginner:** Let the weight of your arm draped over your head slowly stretch the side of your ribcage. **Advanced:** Grab the outside of your foot.

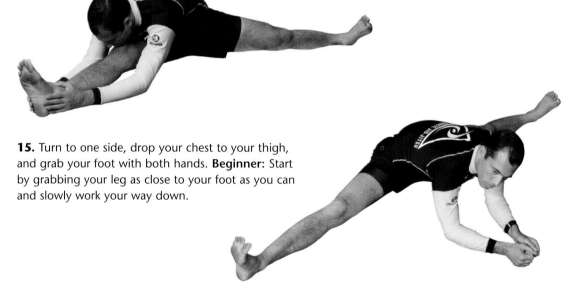

15. Turn to one side, drop your chest to your thigh, and grab your foot with both hands. **Beginner:** Start by grabbing your leg as close to your foot as you can and slowly work your way down.

AGR **16.** Lower your torso toward the ground. Again, beginners will find this very difficult and may start by simply leaning forward and trying to touch their fingertips on the ground. Once you achieve that, start "walking" your hands forward to help lower your torso to the ground.

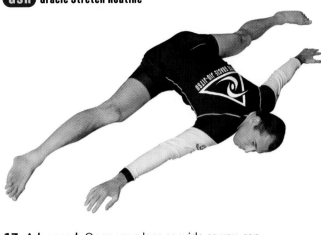

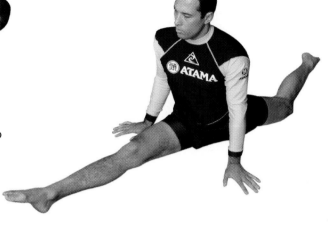

17. Advanced: Open your legs as wide as you can, toes pointing out. Exhale and start to lower your torso (back straight) forward toward the ground. Most people will not have Royce's flexibility and won't be able to go as far as he does here, but it is important to know what your objective is. Most beginners cannot open their legs past 90 degrees and will hardly be able to lower their torso because their hamstrings are tight, but with repetition you will see great improvement, and with a looser hamstring you will also relieve pressure on your lower back, so be sure to practice this stretch. Start by attempting to place your hands on the floor in front of you and then work toward getting your elbows on the floor. See how close you can get your chest to the floor.

AGR **18.** Return to your start position (13) and twist your body to the right. Place your hands on the sides of your body and keep your back straight. Again, beginners should get their legs as wide open as possible.

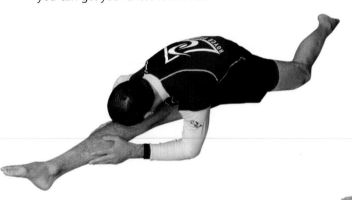

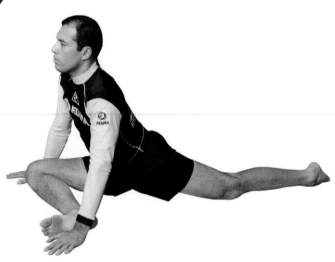

19. While keeping your back as straight as possible, lower your torso toward your right leg until your head touches it. Start slowly and exhale as you bend down. **Beginner:** Grab your leg with your hands to help pull your torso down. Pull down slightly until you feel your hamstring tighten and pause there for a few seconds, exhale and relax. See if you can go a little further, but don't push it!

20. Come back to center and bend your forward leg at your knee so that your lower leg is at 90 degrees. Put your hands down on the floor, head up, and exhale.

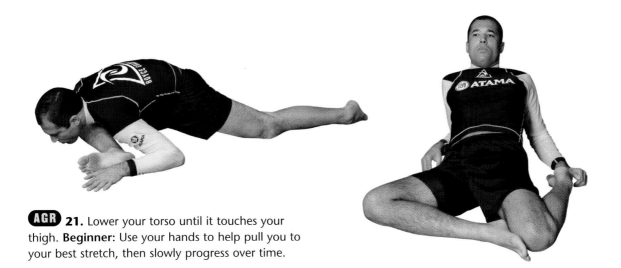

AGR **21.** Lower your torso until it touches your thigh. **Beginner:** Use your hands to help pull you to your best stretch, then slowly progress over time.

AGR **22.** Bring your back leg in and have your forward foot touch your rear knee. Lean back and feel the stretch on your back leg quadriceps. Place your hand on the mat to control the lean. **Advanced:** Go all the way until your back touches the mat.

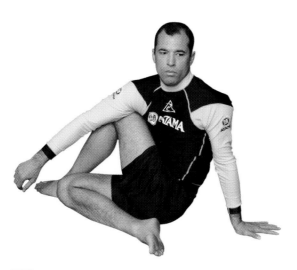

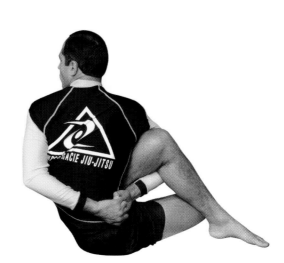

AGR **23.** Loop your left leg over the top of your right leg, placing your foot just outside of your thigh. Get your right arm over your left knee and place your left hand on the mat. Turn your head and torso to the left and stretch your lower back.

AGR **24.** From your previous position, reach your right hand through the gap created by your left leg and grab your left hand behind your back. **Beginner:** Try touching your right hip with your right hand.

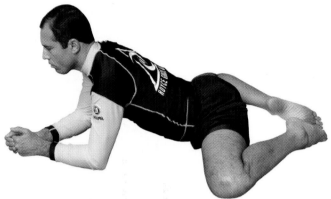

25. Get on all fours and slowly let your knees go out while keeping your feet together. Try getting your pelvis to touch the ground.

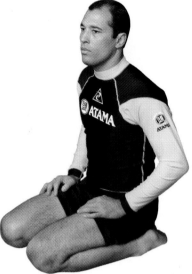

26. Kneel down with your buttocks touching your heels. Keep your head up and your back straight.

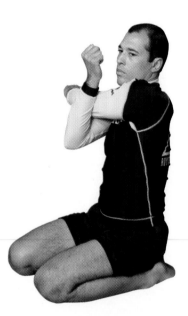

AGR **27.** Reach across with your left arm and hook your right arm behind your left elbow. Use your right arm to help stretch your left shoulder as you pull your left arm to your right. Keep your torso as straight as possible (in other words, try not to rotate your shoulders).

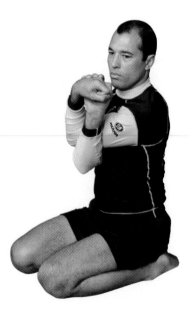

AGR **28.** Bring your forearm up and grab the top outside of your left hand with your right one. Pull your elbows to your chest. Pull your wrist down and outward.

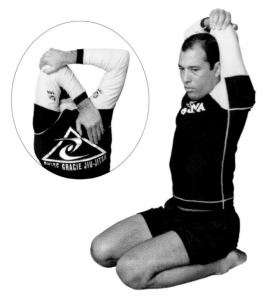

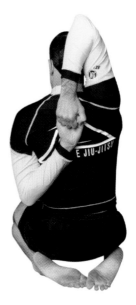

29. Reach back behind your head with your left arm. Reach over your head with your right hand, grab your left elbow, and pull it down and back, stretching your triceps.

AGR **30.** Reach behind your back and under with your left arm. Reach over your head and back with your right arm until your can grab your hands.
Beginner: Use a towel to help connect your hands. Stretch your left triceps and right shoulder.

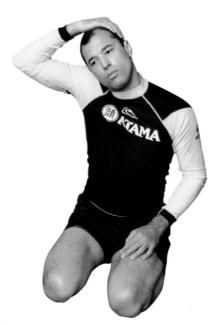

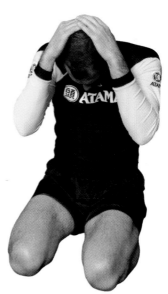

AGR **31.** Kneel on the floor with your buttocks resting on your heels. Place your right hand over your head, grab the left side of your head, and pull it to your right, stretching your neck to the side.

AGR **32.** Place both hands behind your head and pull it forward, stretching your neck.

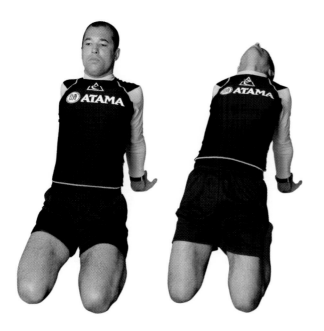

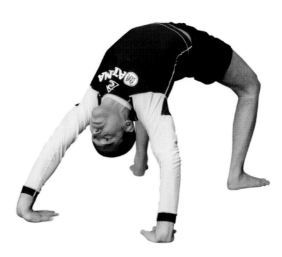

33. Place your hands behind your body. Raise your hips and look back, stretching your shoulders and abdominals.

34. Lie on your back with your heels close to your buttocks. Plant the palms of your hands next to your shoulders and push up, stretching your abdominals.

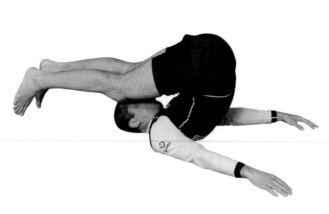

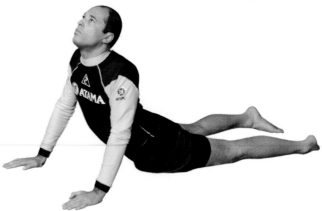

AGR **35.** Lie flat on the floor, face up, arms at your sides. Slowly raise your legs off the floor until they are vertical. Keep your legs straight and continue to lower them until your toes touch the ground. This stretch helps the lower back, neck, and hamstrings. **Beginner:** Make sure you have properly warmed up your neck. Do your stretch on a slightly raised platform so your head hangs over the end. **Advanced:** Put your knees on the ground next to your shoulders.

36. Lie on the mat with your face down. Plant your hands next to your shoulders, push up without lifting your hips off the mat, and look up. This stretches the abs and torso.

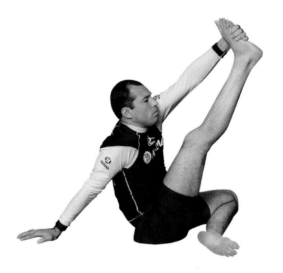

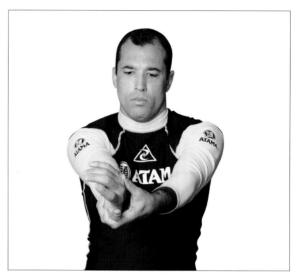

37. Sit on the mat with your left leg curled in front of your body and your right hand flat on the mat for balance. Straighten your right leg out and up while holding the sole of your foot with your left hand, stretching the hamstrings. **Beginner:** Grab the ankle and keep the knee bent. Slowly reach forward with your hand toward your foot and straighten your leg as well.

38. Stands with both arms stretched. Rotate your right palm counterclockwise and use your left hand to assist in stretching the wrist and the elbow.

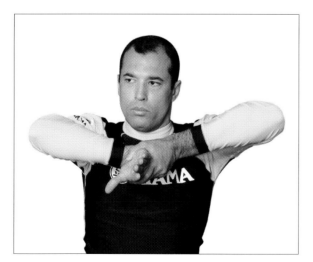

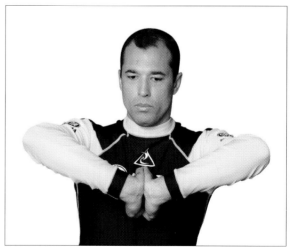

39. Bend your arms at the elbows and continue to stretch your wrist as you rotate your right hand clockwise while assisting with the left one. Notice the thumb hooking over the bottom of the right hand. This stretch isolates the wrist only.

40. Touch both palms together with your fingers facing in and arms bent. Drive your hands forward and away from your body, stretching the fingers.

Two-Person Stretch Routine

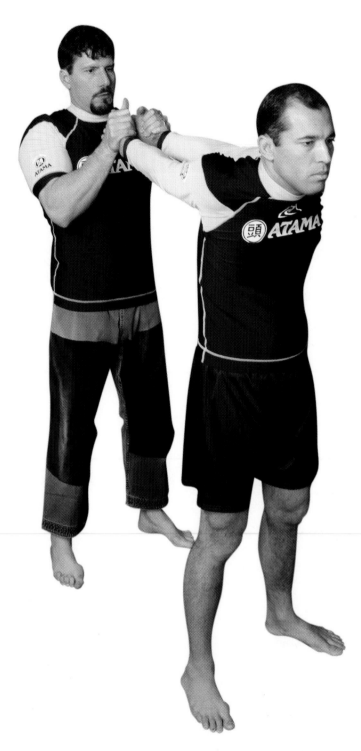

1. Nono grabs both Royce's hands, thumbs up and palms out, and pulls them together behind Royce, stretching the shoulders and chest.

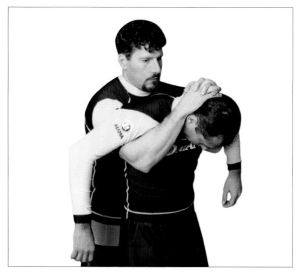

2. Nono reaches under Royce's armpits, locking his hands behind Royce's head, and pushes it down and forward, stretching the back of the neck.

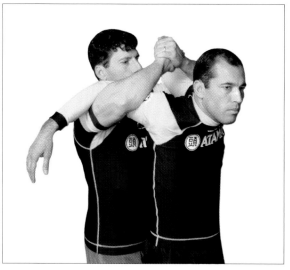

3. Nono then locks his hands so that his elbows are near Royce's biceps and pulls his arms together, stretching the chest and shoulders.

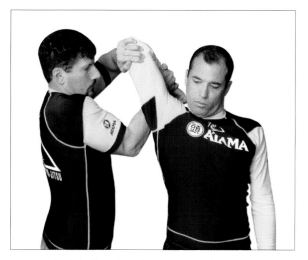

4. Nono's right hand grabs Royce's right wrist and pulls it over Royce's back while his left hand pushes Royce's right elbow back, stretching the triceps and shoulder.

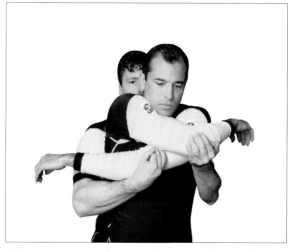

5. Royce stands and crosses his arms in front of his chest. Nono reaches from behind and grabs Royce's elbows with his hands, pulling them further back, stretching the shoulders.

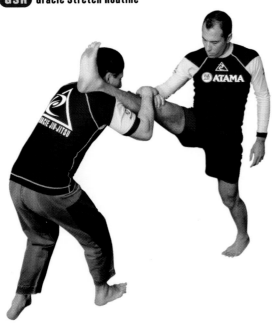

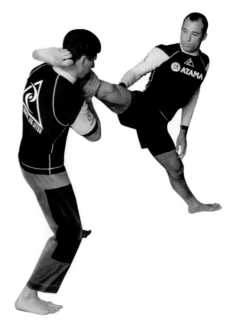

6. Royce places his right leg over Nono's right shoulder while facing him. Nono's hands go on top of Royce's knee to keep the leg straight as he slowly raises his body to increase the stretch on the hamstring. **Beginner:** Start with your partner on his knees and the leg slightly bent. **Advanced:** Continue until you can touch your thigh/knee to your head.

7. Royce places his right leg on Nono's shoulder while sideways to him. Nono's hands go near Royce's knee to keep the leg straight. Royce raises his leg as high as he can. **Beginner:** Start with your partner on his knees or holding your leg with his hands low. **Advanced:** Hold your partner's left hand with your right hand and lift your leg as high as possible. This stretches the groin area (adductors).

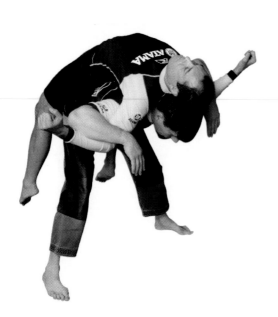

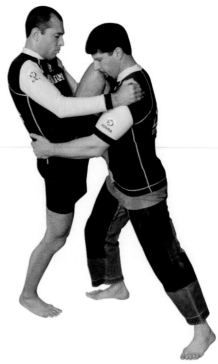

8. Royce begins back-to-back with Nono. Nono interlocks his arms with Royce's arms and bends forward at the waist, lifting Royce off the ground and stretching the shoulders.

9. Royce place's his left shin on Nono's chest as he leans forward, pushing the leg to Royce's chest. This stretches the hips and hamstrings. **Beginner:** Start with your leg at 90 degrees.

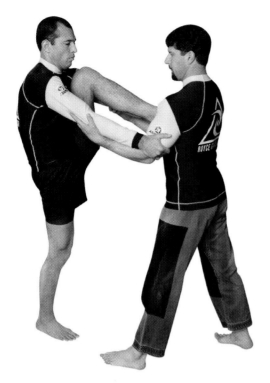

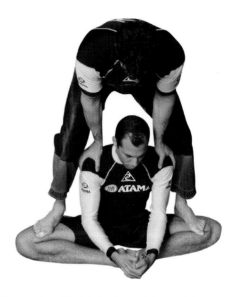

10. Advanced: Place your foot on the spotter's chest as he pushes forward. Try touching your knee to your chest.

11. Royce sits with his back straight and feet touching while Nono stands with each foot on top of Royce's thighs, stretching the adductors (groin area).
Beginner: Have your partner face you and push down on your knees with his hands for the stretch.

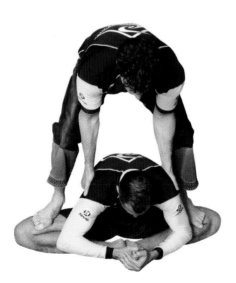

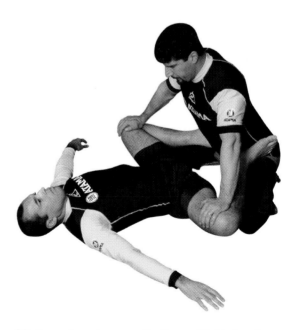

12. Advanced: Lean forward with your torso until you can touch your face to the floor.

13. Royce lays down on the floor with his legs bent at the knees while Nono pushes down on the knees to stretch the groin area.

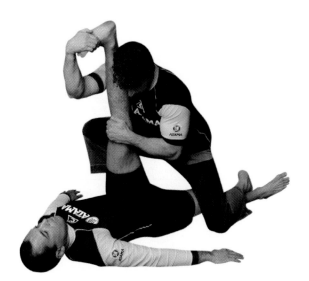

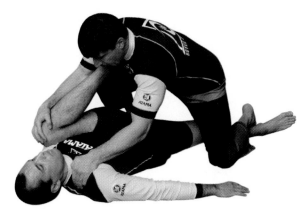

14. Royce lies on the mat with his right leg straight on the floor while Nono pushes Royce's left leg toward his head, stretching the hamstring.
Beginner: Keep your right knee bent to ease the stretch. **Advanced:** Pull your knee to your face/chest.

15. Royce lies on the floor with his right leg straight and places his left foot on Nono's chest. Nono traps Royce's right leg with his shin to keep it from lifting as he pushes forward, driving Royce's knee to his chest. He may go through a range of motion, circling the leg.

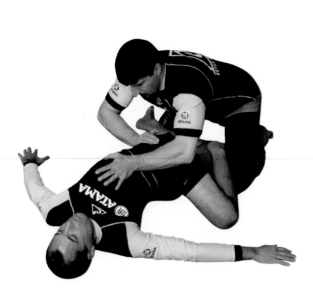

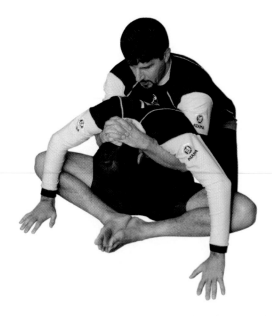

16. Royce lies on the mat with both legs bent at the knee and twists his hips so that his left leg is over the right one. Nono pushes on Royce's chest with his left hand, keeping Royce's back on the ground while he pushes Royce's left hip with his right hand to stretch the hips and lower back.

17. Royce sits with his back straight, legs bent, and feet touching. Nono wraps his arms under Royce's arms, interlocking his fingers behind Royce's neck. As he straightens his arms, Nono stretches Royce's neck and back.

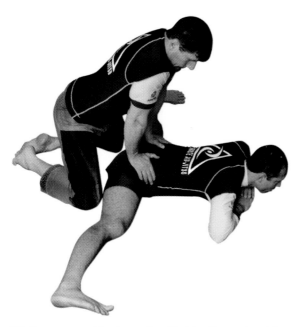

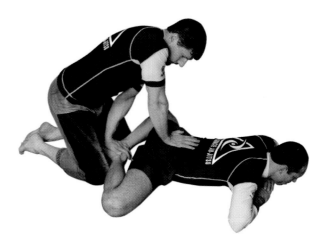

18. Royce is on his stomach with his elbows touching the mat and his legs open as wide as possible. Nono pushes down on his hips to stretch the groin area. **Beginner:** Start with your legs bent at the knee. **Advanced:** Spread your legs out until your hips touch the ground.

19. Continuing with the same stretch, Royce brings his feet together as Nono locks them on the floor with his left hand and pushes down on Royce's hips with his right one.

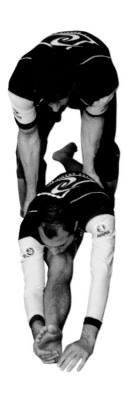

20. Royce starts doing the splits with both legs spread, one in front and one in back, as he reaches to touch his right toes with his hands. Nono pushes down on Royce's back to help the hamstring stretch. **Beginner:** Start by kneeling on the mat with your arms straight and palms on the ground. Begin the stretch by straightening your front leg first, then your back leg as you balance your weight on your arms.

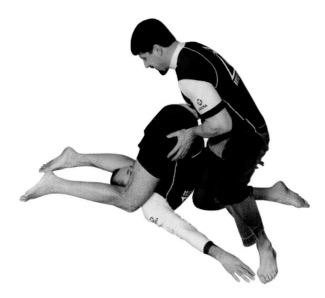

21. This stretch is a two-person version of stretch 35 in the GSR. Royce lies flat on the floor, face up, arms at his sides, and slowly raises his legs off the floor until they are vertical. He keeps his legs straight and continues to lower them until the toes touch the ground. Nono is on his knees and presses down and back on Royce's hips to accentuate the stretch. This stretch works the lower back, neck, and hamstrings.

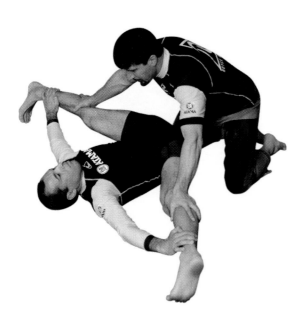

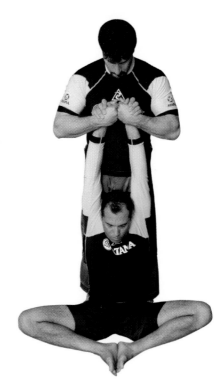

22. Royce opens his legs wide and places his back on the mat as Nono presses down on Royce's calves so his knees and toes touch the mat, stretching his hips and hamstrings.

23. Royce starts sitting down with his back straight and legs bent at the knees, the soles of his feet touching. Nono grabs Royce's hands and pulls his arms up, stretching the shoulders and elongating the spine.

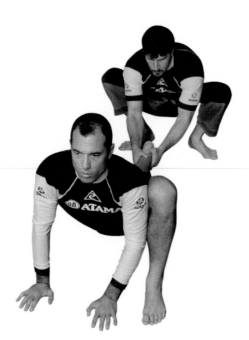

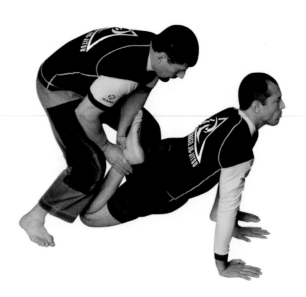

24. Royce starts in a pushup position, arms in front and legs straight back. He takes a step forward with his left leg so that his left foot is just outside his left hand. Nono grabs Royce's right ankle and pulls it back, accentuating the adductors and quadriceps.

25. Continuing from that position, Nono pushes Royce's right foot toward his buttocks, stretching the quadriceps even more.

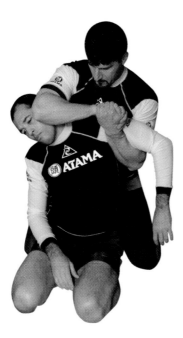

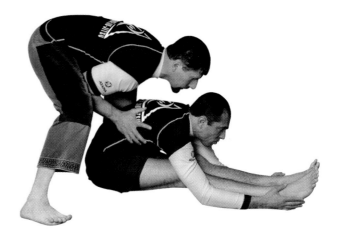

26. Royce kneels on the mat with his torso straight. Nono hooks his left arm under Royce's left arm and locks his hands together with his right arm at 90 degrees. Nono's triceps pushes on Royce's head to stretch the neck.

27. Royce sits with both legs straight ahead of him and lowers his torso, touching his hands to his toes. Nono helps the stretch by pushing down and forward on Royce's back. Nono starts by pushing on Royce's shoulders and, as Royce feels comfortable and lowers his torso, Nono will drop his hands toward Royce's lower back, pushing Royce's back toward his legs.

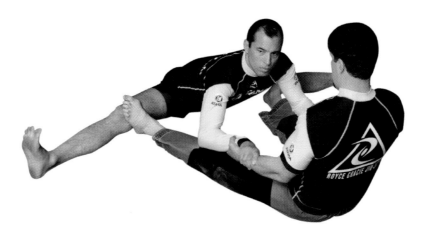

28. Royce sits on the mat with both legs open and straight. Nono is facing him with his feet pushing on Royce's thighs and their hands interlocked. Nono will lean back as he pulls Royce's torso forward and at the same time pushes Royce's legs open, stretching the adductors.

The Exercises

All martial arts exercises are complex moves that require most of the muscle groups in the body to perform in a coordinated fashion. Therefore, it is important to develop your muscles not only to be strong but also to be able to function in different planes of motion. The key is not simply muscle power but functional muscle power—the ability to deliver power in a rapidly changing environment. For example, a person who has trained strictly for power may be able to squat a tremendous amount of weight under perfect conditions in the gym. In a judo match, however, he wouldn't have the luxury of setting up for perfect form, and he may be unable to deliver the power needed for the throw. An athlete with the proper martial arts training, on the other hand, should be able to adapt to the unpredictability of a match and be able to deliver power in less than ideal situations while still remaining in control of his actions and without injuring himself. That is *functional* muscle power, and it is what these exercises are designed to give you.

We are proud of the fact that the *Superfit* system emphasizes you, rather than specialized equipment. Anyone can take this book, make a few basic purchases, go in their garage, and do the workouts. With some dumbbells, a barbell, a jump rope, and some tubing, you can kick ass.

Breathing During the Exercises

Breathing is the most basic function of life. You can go a month without food or a couple of days without water, but more than a minute without oxygen and you are toast! Providing the muscles and brain with a rich supply of oxygen is essential in the martial arts, where the constant movement and stress tax the body, creating the need to learn to breathe properly. If you learn to breathe correctly during the exercises, your

If You Are Purchasing Equipment

Tips for Building Your Superfit Home Gym

Start small! You need some space dedicated to working out, the basic equipment listed below, this book, and motivation. That's it. To get yourself going as quickly and efficiently as possible, do these things:

- Consider your goals. Because martial arts training is multidimensional, the Superfit program uses several simple types of equipment to make you fast, flexible, and powerful. To begin, you don't need a bunch of weights, tubes, or plyoballs, but you do need to be able to execute all the exercises. Get the basics and get started!

- Consider your space. Whether you plan to work out in your garage or your living room, you'll need room enough for stretching and ceilings high enough for jumping rope. Carpet will slow you down. Available space may influence your decision between fixed and solid weights.

- Consider your budget. Each item listed below can be had inexpensively, but—as with most things—you get what you pay for in exercise equipment. If your budget is limited, we recommend buying fewer pieces of good quality equipment

and building as you can. A word to the wise: It pays to shop around!

- Look for hassle-free equipment. You want to be training, not fooling around with gear! Don't underestimate the value of customer service reps at specialty equipment stores. They are your best source of information in finding exactly the right equipment for you.

The Basics

If you prefer the convenience of working out at home, you'll need to purchase a few pieces of equipment. At minimum, you'll need:

a flat bench
a barbell
a dumbbell set
elastic tubing or a weight vest
a jump rope
medicine balls
weight plates (if you use adjustable
  free weights)

When looking at flat benches, keep stability in mind. A basic 36-inch bench with 2-inch tubing will provide all the durability and security you can ask for. More expensive benches are adjustable, opening up your workout routines to include incline exercises.

If You Are Purchasing Equipment

Free weights come in two varieties: fixed (also called solid) and adjustable (or pro-style). Fixed weights involve much less hassle as you switch from one exercise to another, but they are more expensive and can take up a great deal more room. If space is limited, we recommend going with a standard set of adjustable weights, which usually includes two dumbbell bars, a 5- or 6-foot barbell bar, weight clips, and around 110 lbs. of plates. At the very least, you'll want a few 2.5 lb. plates, a couple at 5 lbs., and a couple at 10 lbs. Broad, flat endcaps with permanent weight markings, although not necessary, will make your life a lot easier, and hex bolts fasten more securely than Allen bolts.

Elastic tubing is measured by the outside diameter and ranges from 1/8" to 1". You'll need to experiment a little to determine what works best for you, but we recommend that you start at least with the 1/4" tube and double it if you need extra power in the beginning. As you advance, you will need thicker tubes that you may have to double or triple, depending on your size and strength. As in selecting free weights, apply the rule of thumb that you need the load that will allow you to get through each exercise set but make you struggle on the last repetition.

Medicine balls (also called plyoballs or body balls) come in leather, rubber, polyurethane, and vinyl. They are available in increments of 1 or 2 lbs., which gives you great versatility in choosing and increasing your load. Those that are filled with air or gel bounce when thrown against the ground or a wall, which can be very useful if you are training by yourself. Unlike free weights, medicine balls allow you to move in three dimensions, not only rotating, flexing, and extending, but also replicating explosive motions like throwing punches. These same benefits can create problems, so start slowly with a light medicine ball (between 4 and 8 lbs.) until you understand the power that they can develop. For grip strength, consider a 2 lb. ball.

Resources

Dumbbells, weights, and benches are best purchased at specialty exercise stores like Sportmart, Sports Authority, or Gart Brothers.

Elastics for the power series exercises can be found at scuba dive shops (they are used on spearguns) or at places like:

www.jumpusa.com *or* **www.reefscuba.com**

Harnesses (if you decide to purchase them) can be ordered from:

www.jumpusa.com

Medicine Balls can be ordered from www.jumpusa.com or through:

Century Martial Arts products

(www.centuryma.com)

ability will become apparent in your training and competing as well. The opposite is also true: improper breathing during workouts almost ensures ineffective breath in competition. Too often we see people simply inhale and try to retain the breath during an intense period of fighting, only to release the air all at once and be exhausted. In general, the correct way to breathe during exercising is as follows: *inhale* prior to the exertion, then *exhale* as you push the weight or deliver the punch. Take a breath before you exert any energy and exhale as you exert it.

Different Exercises and Their Purposes

To develop your functional muscle power, the *Superfit* system employs six types of exercises: abdominal, cardiovascular, free weight, isolateral, plyometric, and the Power Series. Each type of exercise is designed to work a particular part of the body or to prepare you for a particular aspect of martial art competition.

As we explain in greater detail later, the *Superfit* system encourages you to experiment by altering the workouts. This will prevent them from becoming stale and ensure that you stay focused and challenged. To help you modify the workouts, each exercise in the workout routines is marked with an icon that refers to the categories of exercises below. Using the icons, you can easily replace exercises from one category with others from the same category, giving you great flexibility without any guesswork!

Let's take a few minutes to consider each category of exercise.

AB Abdominal

In the martial arts, as in other highly physical performance sports such as gymnastics, explosiveness, speed, and power come ultimately from your center—your abdominals. Whether positioning your body to execute a technique, striking with your arms or legs, or blocking, parrying, or absorbing a blow, your abdominal strength is critical to your effectiveness. A rock-hard midsection not only gives you the advantage of stability as you move, but it also protects the most vulnerable part of your body. Special attention given to conditioning your abs will pay off in greater performance and increased protection.

Our workouts challenge you to work your abs every day you exercise. But don't think we expect you just to grit your teeth through an endless number of crunches. We've provided a range of exercises that will keep you interested, keep you challenged, and make your midsection the powerful, elastic core martial artists need.

CC Cardiovascular Conditioning

Cardiovascular exercises increase your ability to pump blood and process oxygen. Typically, they involve low-impact, large-muscle movement over a sustained period of time, which raises your heart rate to 50 percent of its maximum level or above. Examples of cardiovascular exercises include running, walking, stair climbing, and swimming. Benefits from cardiovascular exercise include lowering blood pressure, increasing HDL (good) cholesterol, decreasing LDL (bad) cholesterol, along with increased heart and lung function and efficiency and decreased anxiety, tension, and depression. The National Institute on Aging states, "endurance activities help prevent or delay many diseases that seem to come with age. In some cases, endurance activity can also improve chronic diseases or their symptoms." Cardiovascular capacity is not only a major component of feeling good and being healthy, it is also vital for the martial artist. If you tire during a competition or a fight, you are doomed. There is a saying in the Brazilian jiu-jitsu circles: "A tired man is a dead man!" If your body cannot process the oxygen necessary to meet the physical demands of fighting and to keep your mind sharp, then your fight is over!

In 1994, in his third fight of the night, 175-pound Royce fought the 262-pounder, Dan "The Beast" Severn, in UFC 4 for over 15 nonstop minutes. In 2000, Royce fought Japanese fighter Kasushi Sakuraba for an incredible 90 minutes (six 15-minute rounds). And all that time, Royce was thinking clearly and ready to fight even longer. Of course, no one expects you to be able to fight so long, but the point is that your ability to perform is directly related to your cardiovascular conditioning.

FW Free Weights

Machines are very stable and are good for the development of specific muscles, but they don't imitate real life very well. When you use a barbell, however, you introduce an element of instability that engages different muscles. When you go one step further and introduce dumbbells in each hand, you increase the instability factor and make it even more difficult to balance and control the weights. This accomplishes two things:

First, you develop your "stabilizers" and "neutralizers." These are two groups of muscles whose objective is to balance and control. Many athletes develop very strong muscles, but unless they have equally capable neutralizers and stabilizers, they will develop joint problems because their joints cannot withstand their newly acquired power. This risk is amplified by the rigor of martial arts training, which demands maximum ranges of both power and motion in the joints.

Second, using free weights develops your motor coordination and challenges your brain to stay in the exercise. When you exercise with a machine, the axis and steel of the machine allow the weight to move only in a prescribed manner; therefore, you can exercise almost without engaging your brain. With the free weights, you must always maintain focus on your actions or you may lose control of the weight. This causes you to tire more quickly, but challenging your body with these additional variables stimulates and trains your muscles, as well as your neuromuscular system, to perform better and longer.

Another problem with training on machines is that you may not find the equipment you are used to or need for your specific program when you are traveling or fighting in another city or country. Every gym, however, has dumbbells and barbells, and it's easy enough to pack a rope and some elastic wherever you go. When Royce is in Japan for fights, he doesn't worry about whether the hotel gym has the proper machines or whether he needs to find a special gym to work out, because all he needs are the basic things found in even the most humble gym.

You may notice that we have nonetheless included two machine exercises: the machine cross and the machine uppercut. These exercises can dramatically increase martial artists' punching power and can best be done with machines. If you don't have access to machines, don't worry. Our workouts will still optimize your punch. If you do have access to machines, be sure to give exercises 64 and 65 a try. You'll feel their impact immediately.

ISO Isolaterals

Isolaterals are exercises designed to balance your muscular structure. Typically, they involve working one limb or one side of the body at a time while performing conventional exercises like the bench press, military press, or upright row. In the bench press with dumbbells, for example, you would hold one weight steady in one hand while performing the exercise with weight in the other.

The *Superfit* system involves doing a number of isolateral repetitions to one side and then changing sides and repeating the routine on the other side—not necessarily for the same number of repetitions. This balances your muscle power. Since most people have a dominant side, isolateral exercises can be adjusted to create balance. For instance, if your right side is dominant, you can do 10 reps on the right and 15 on the left. This will give you greater ability to react and execute moves to both sides. Most martial artists have a tendency to do moves better to one side, be it the kata that you can only perform going to your right or the guard pass that you are only comfortable doing to the left. Any such "blind side" will be exploited by a skilled adversary. Isolaterals close up such weaknesses.

PL Plyometrics

The *Superfit* system uses quite a few exercises that involve plyometrics— quick bursts that repeatedly stretch and contract your muscles. Plyometric exercises are perfect for the martial arts because they connect explosive movement with power and strength, enhancing your ability to perform under realistic conditions. By training your body to move with quickness and agility, you will gain both. As exercise guru Paul Chek likes to point out, "Train slow, be slow!"

Being able to deliver power at the precise instant in an active environment is exactly what martial artists require. Take, for instance, a wrestler attempting to execute a takedown. First, he coils his body in anticipation of the attack, then he lunges forward at his opponent until he secures the proper grip. At that instant, he must be able to switch once again to using power and speed to take the opponent down.

If you concentrate simply on specific aerobic conditioning and weight training exercises, you are only preparing yourself to endure and to apply power in a static environment, which is the furthest thing from the realities of fighting. In fighting, you are required not only to have stamina and strength, but also to be able to react to the opportunities or demands that arise during a match against a living, thinking opponent. Plyometrics are the key to developing such "reactionary instincts" in your muscles.

In this book you will be shown a variety of plyometric exercises such as the box jumps (66), the lateral jumps (68), and some of the medicine ball exercises. Typically in plyometrics, one attempts to perform the greatest number of repetitions in a set period of time without losing form. For that reason these exercises not only challenge your explosion and coordination but they also increase your stamina and endurance.

A word of caution: plyometrics are high-impact exercises and as such they may aggravate conditions such as tendonitis, arthritis, and bursitis. Make sure you maintain proper form while doing plyometrics. If you begin to tire and lose form, stop immediately. If you practice after your form is lost, you will only be training yourself to execute improper techniques. Losing form is your signal to take a break.

PS Power Series

The *Superfit* power series exercises are power-building exercises that take plyometrics to the next level. Like plyometrics, the power series typically (with some exceptions like the static wall sit) involve a quick, explosive movement, and the key to the exercises is to begin with little or no pressure and concentrate on form, explosion, and speed. What you want is to do the greatest number of repetitions in a certain amount of time without compromising technique. If you start to lose form, stop.

What distinguishes the power series exercises is their unique attention to combining cardiovascular fitness and muscular strength while replicating real-life movements vital for martial artists—lateral motions and explosive motions like punches, kicks, and jumps. To achieve this combination, many of the exercises involve the use of a harness and elastic cords (or a weight vest) to create progressive resistance. As you master each exercise and reach reasonable speed, increase your resistance or have your spotter add pressure. You'll increase your endurance and your strength at the same time.

ABDOMINALS AB

1. Bench Crunches

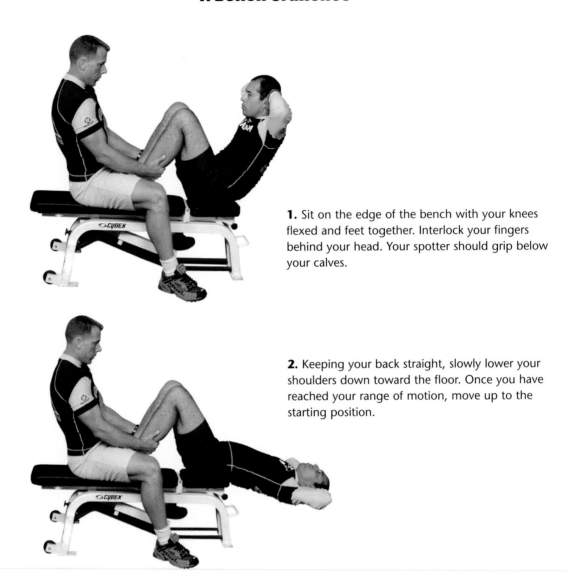

1. Sit on the edge of the bench with your knees flexed and feet together. Interlock your fingers behind your head. Your spotter should grip below your calves.

2. Keeping your back straight, slowly lower your shoulders down toward the floor. Once you have reached your range of motion, move up to the starting position.

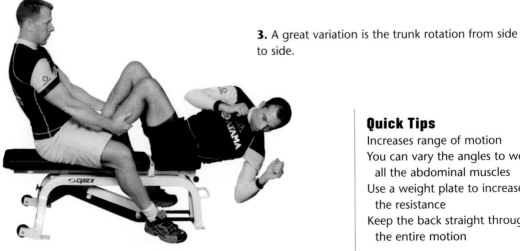

3. A great variation is the trunk rotation from side to side.

Quick Tips
Increases range of motion
You can vary the angles to work
  all the abdominal muscles
Use a weight plate to increase
  the resistance
Keep the back straight through
  the entire motion

2. Medicine Ball Stand-Ups

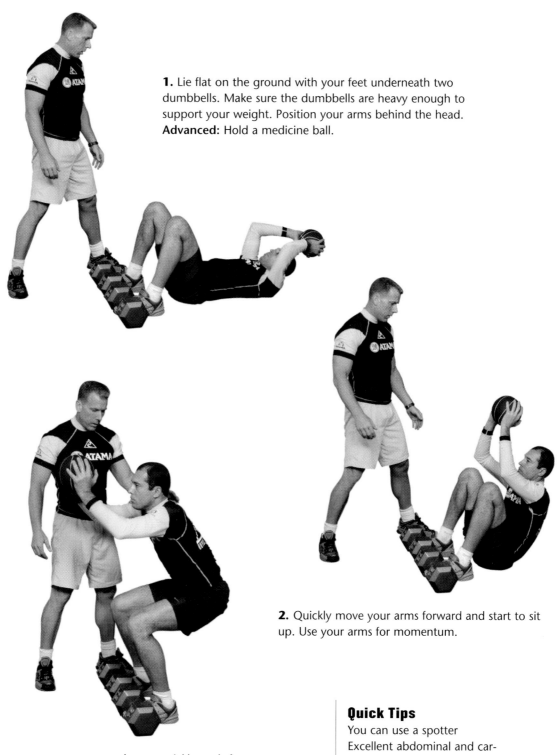

1. Lie flat on the ground with your feet underneath two dumbbells. Make sure the dumbbells are heavy enough to support your weight. Position your arms behind the head. **Advanced:** Hold a medicine ball.

2. Quickly move your arms forward and start to sit up. Use your arms for momentum.

3. Once your arms pass your knees, quickly push forward with your legs, moving into a standing position.

Quick Tips

You can use a spotter

Excellent abdominal and cardiovascular exercise

Use your arms for momentum to help raise yourself

3. Roll-Ups—Abdominal

1. Position yourself flat on the ground with your arms at your sides. Your feet are off the ground with the knees bent. **Advanced:** Squeeze a medicine ball between your knees for greater resistance.

Quick Tips
Great way to strengthen the lower back

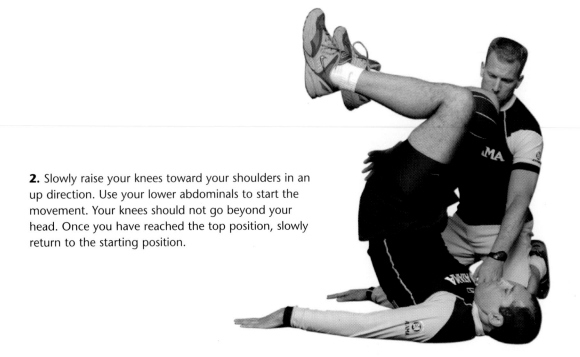

2. Slowly raise your knees toward your shoulders in an up direction. Use your lower abdominals to start the movement. Your knees should not go beyond your head. Once you have reached the top position, slowly return to the starting position.

4. Wheels

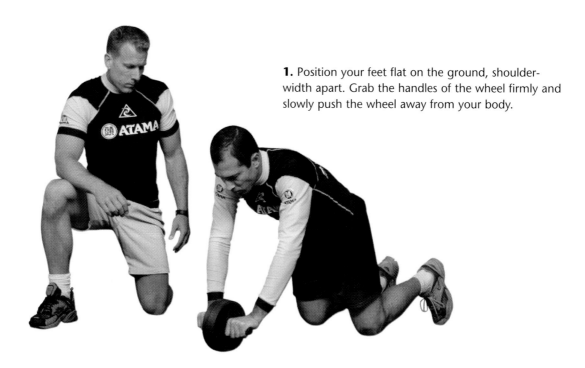

1. Position your feet flat on the ground, shoulder-width apart. Grab the handles of the wheel firmly and slowly push the wheel away from your body.

Quick Tips

Good for both abdominals and lower
  back strength
Good for shoulders and lats
Intermediate/Advanced
Use a weight plate in front of you to
  limit your range of motion

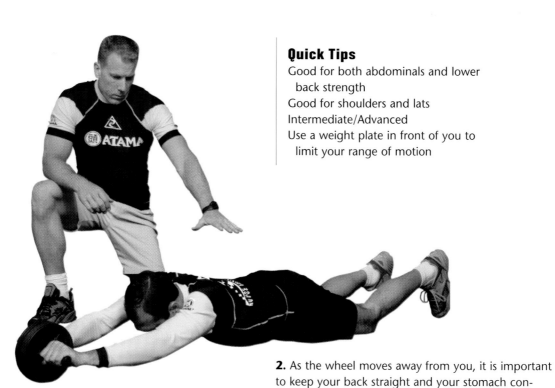

2. As the wheel moves away from you, it is important to keep your back straight and your stomach contracted. Once you have reached your desired range of motion, return to the starting position.

5. Side-to-Side Reaches

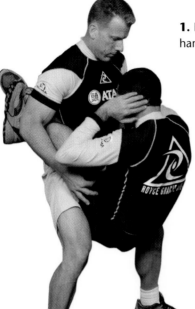

1. Lock your legs around the spotter with your hands behind your head.

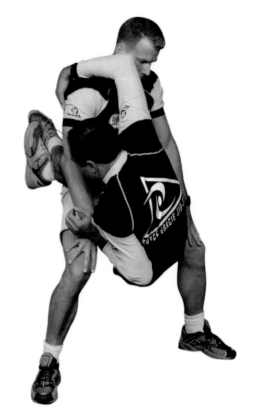

2. Using your abdominals to keep you up, reach across with your right arm and touch the back of the spotter's right shoulder.

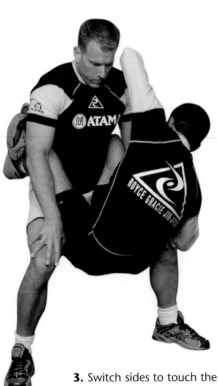

3. Switch sides to touch the left shoulder.

— PART TWO —

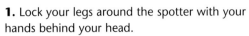

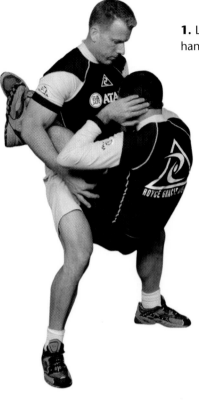

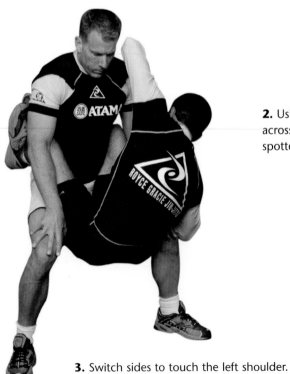

3. Switch sides to touch the left shoulder.

Variation:

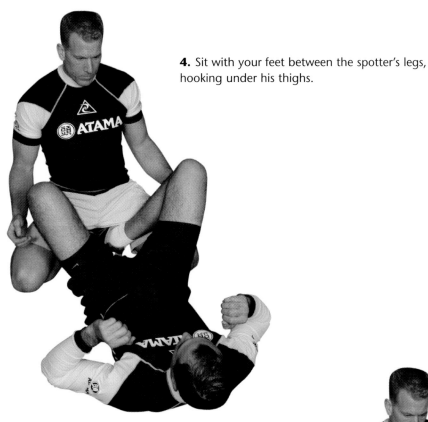

4. Sit with your feet between the spotter's legs, hooking under his thighs.

Quick Tips
Great total body exercise
Develops endurance
Keep the upper-body swing to
  a minimum

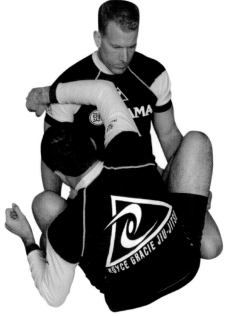

5. Sit up as you reach and touch the back of the spotter's shoulder. Go back down and alternate sides.

6. V-Ups

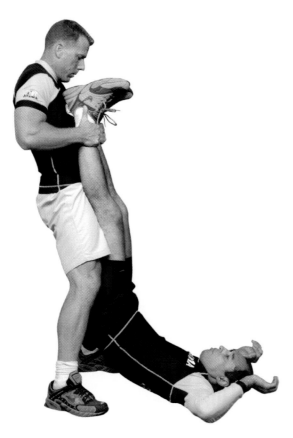

1. Lie flat on the ground with your legs extended up. Arms are bent and parallel to your head. Make sure your spotter's grip is firm!

Quick Tips
Must have a spotter
Good for lower back as well as abs
Intermediate/Advanced

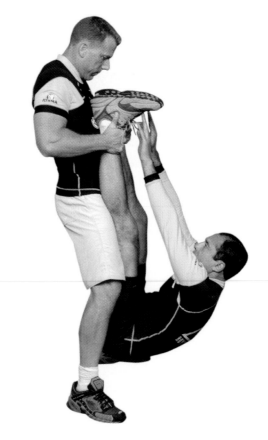

2. Using your abdominals, pull yourself up. As you are moving up, reach with your hands and touch your toes. Slowly lower yourself to the starting position.

Variations:

Variation One: 1. Lie flat on your back and create a V position with your legs. Using your abdominals, lift your shoulders off the floor, touching your hand to the opposite foot, and repeat to the other side.

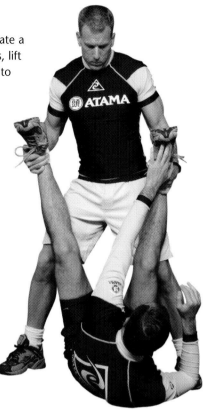

Variation Two: 1. Lock your legs around the spotter and position your hands behind your head.

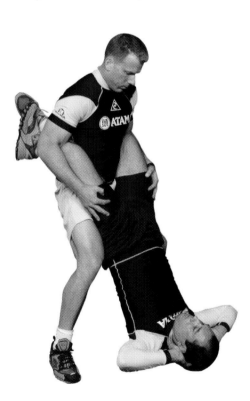

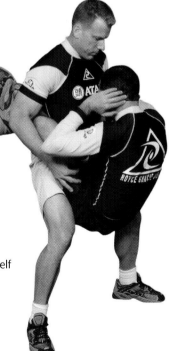

2. Using your abdominals, pull yourself up. Slowly lower yourself to the starting position.

CARDIOVASCULAR CONDITIONING CC

7. Jump Rope

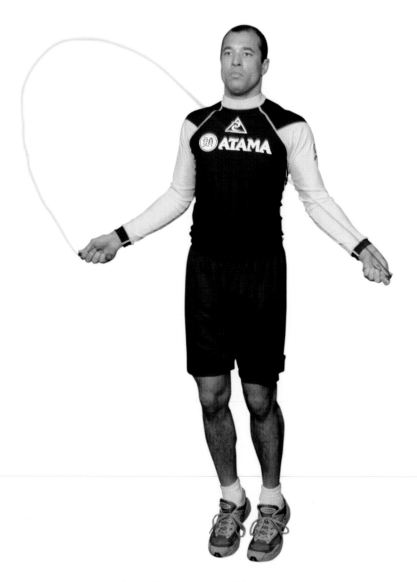

1. Beginner: Start with both feet together and jump rope in place.

2. Intermediate: Every third jump, try to jump extra high through the rope.

Quick Tips
Great endurance exercise
Good for coordination

3. Advanced: Get on a squat stance and continue to jump rope.

8. Lateral Cone Touches

1. Place a pair of cones at least six feet from each other. With your feet shoulder-width apart, bend at the knees and touch the top of the cone.

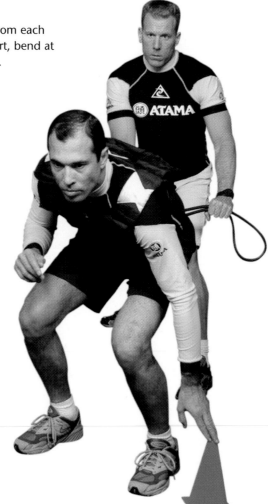

Quick Tips

Great for balance and explosive strength

Great for endurance and agility

Use a weight vest instead of the bungee if no spotter is available

Use different distances and thicknesses of bungee cord to vary the resistance

Concentrate on form and speed. If form suffers, stop the exercise and rest

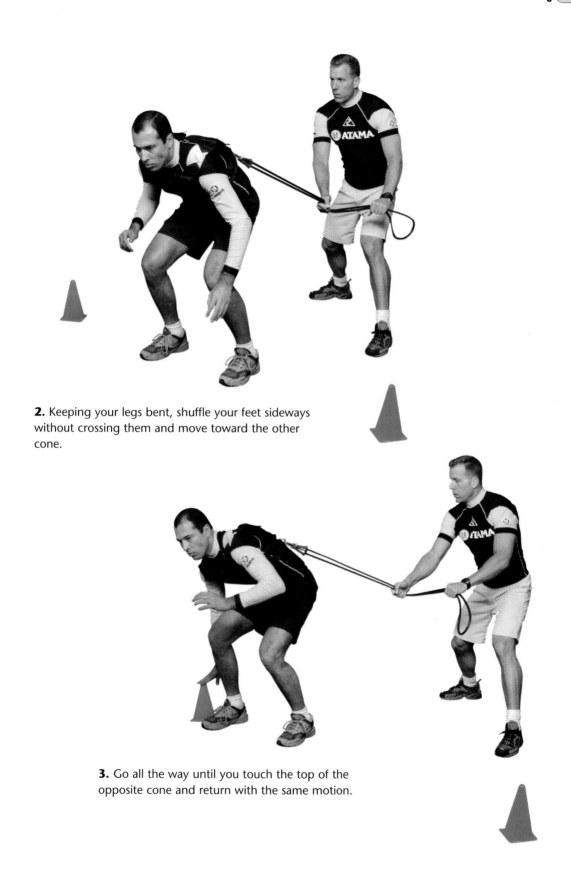

2. Keeping your legs bent, shuffle your feet sideways without crossing them and move toward the other cone.

3. Go all the way until you touch the top of the opposite cone and return with the same motion.

9. Run in Place

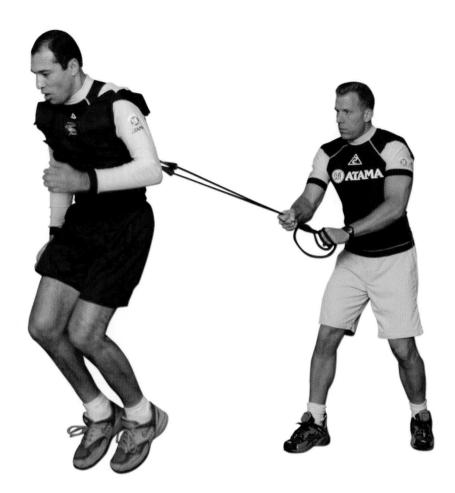

1. Run in place while your spotter controls the pressure.

10. Run and Hold

Same as running in place but spotter lets you run for a certain number of yards, then holds you in place for a set number of seconds.

Quick Tips
Great for balance and explosive strength
Great for endurance and agility
Use a weight vest instead of the bungee if no spotter is available
Use different distances and thicknesses of bungee cord to vary the resistance
Concentrate on form and speed. If form suffers, stop the exercise and rest

11. Soft Sand Run

Run in soft sand for specified length of time. If running on sand is not an option, run in grass for upper limit of time specified. If grass is not an option, see 12.

12. Steady Run or Jog

Run or jog for specified length of time.

13. Sprints

Sprint specified distance at 70–80% intensity unless otherwise noted. Walk or jog back to starting place.

FREE WEIGHTS FW

14. Bench Press—Barbell

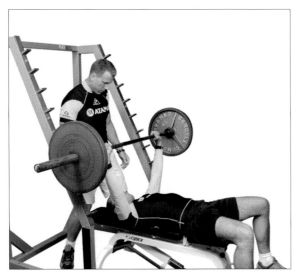

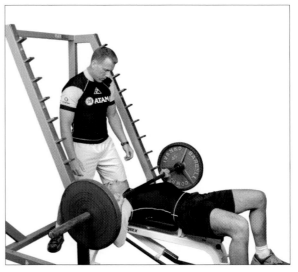

Start/finish: Your grip should be equal, elbows straight and shoulders and buttocks touching the bench. Your feet are flat on the floor.

Midpoint: The descent of the bar is controlled. The bar should gently touch your sternum as you prepare to press the barbell back to the starting position.

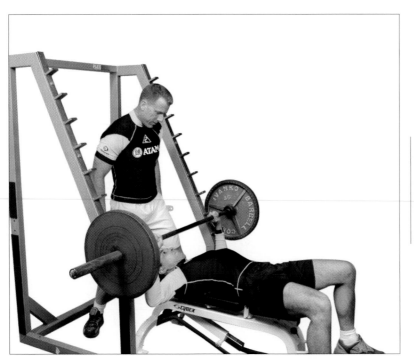

Detail: Keeping your feet and buttocks firmly planted, push the barbell back to the starting position.

QUICK TIPS
Slightly arch your lower back
Always keep your buttocks on
  the bench
Use a spotter

15. Bench Press—Dumbbell

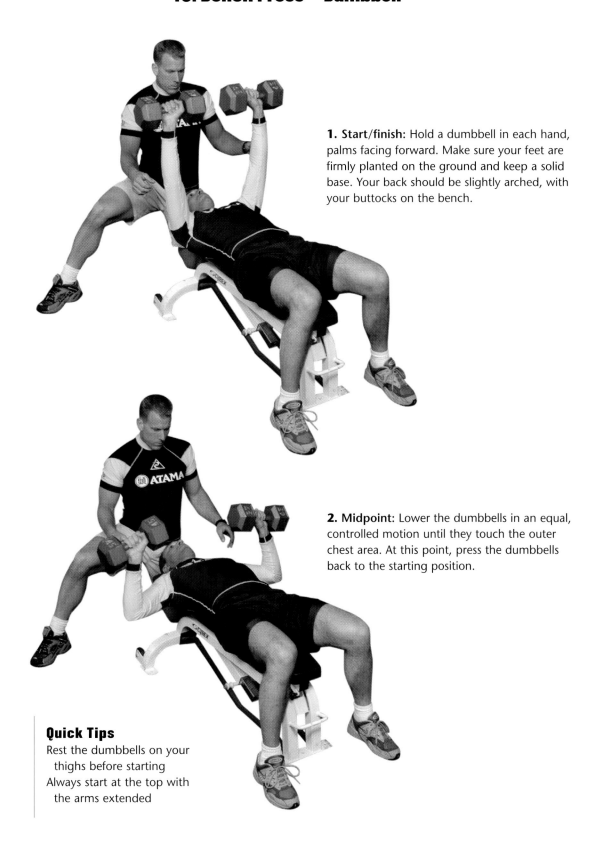

1. Start/finish: Hold a dumbbell in each hand, palms facing forward. Make sure your feet are firmly planted on the ground and keep a solid base. Your back should be slightly arched, with your buttocks on the bench.

2. Midpoint: Lower the dumbbells in an equal, controlled motion until they touch the outer chest area. At this point, press the dumbbells back to the starting position.

Quick Tips
Rest the dumbbells on your
  thighs before starting
Always start at the top with
  the arms extended

16. Bench Press—Narrow Grip Barbell

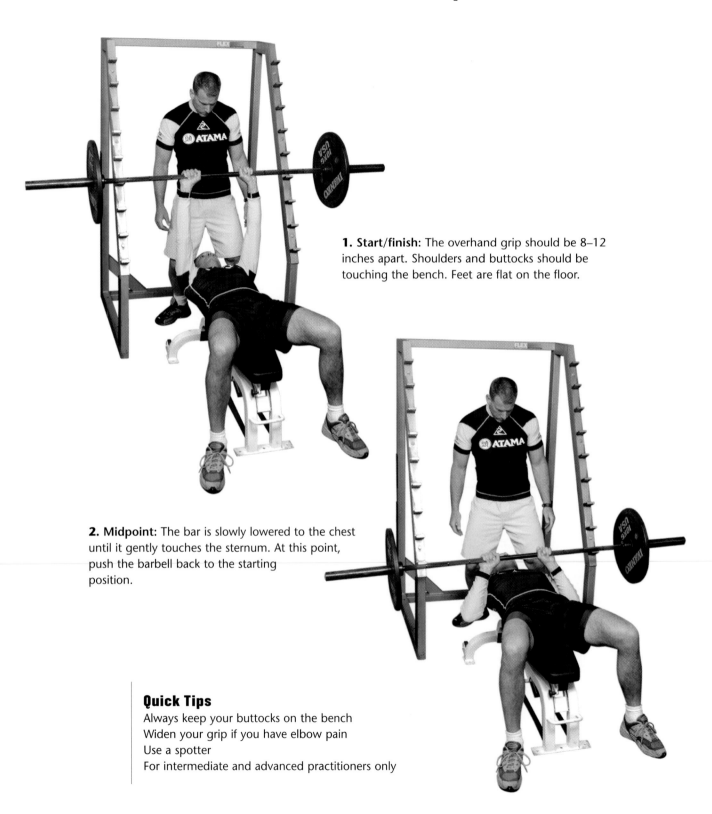

1. Start/finish: The overhand grip should be 8–12 inches apart. Shoulders and buttocks should be touching the bench. Feet are flat on the floor.

2. Midpoint: The bar is slowly lowered to the chest until it gently touches the sternum. At this point, push the barbell back to the starting position.

Quick Tips

Always keep your buttocks on the bench
Widen your grip if you have elbow pain
Use a spotter
For intermediate and advanced practitioners only

17. Front Raise—Barbell

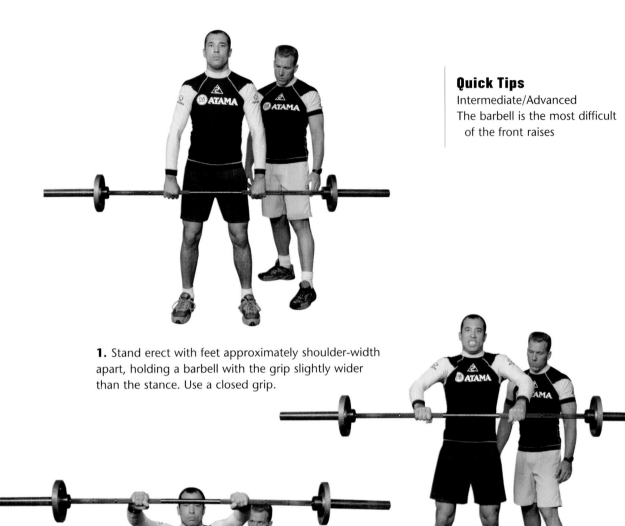

Quick Tips
Intermediate/Advanced
The barbell is the most difficult
  of the front raises

1. Stand erect with feet approximately shoulder-width apart, holding a barbell with the grip slightly wider than the stance. Use a closed grip.

2. Use the arms to raise the barbell, not the legs.

3. Raise the barbell to eye level, then slowly return to the starting position.

18. Front Raise—Dumbbell

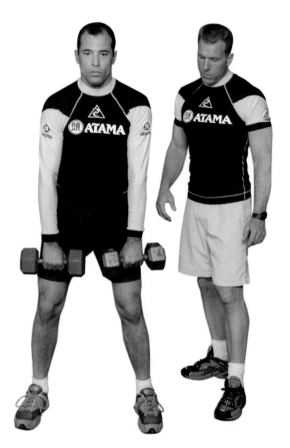

1. Stand erect with feet shoulder-width apart, holding a dumbbell in each hand.

Quick Tips
Great exercise to strengthen the anterior deltoid

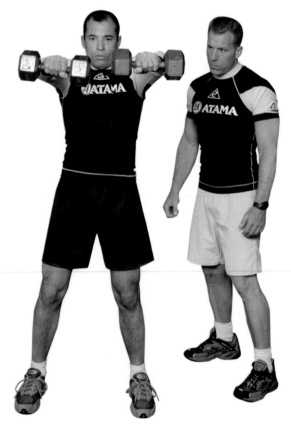

2. Raise the dumbbell to eye level. Hold for 1–2 seconds at the top end, then slowly return to the starting position.

19. Front Raise—Plate

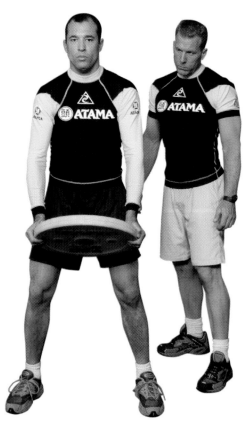

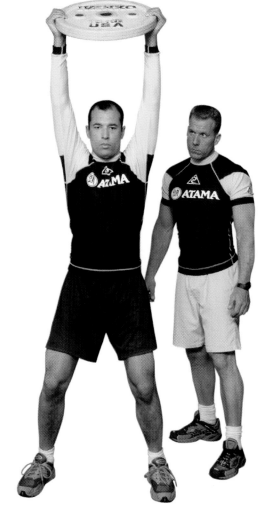

1. Stand erect with feet approximately shoulder-width apart, holding a plate. A plate is a good variation for the front raise, because the weight is more concentrated, challenging the core control in a different manner. The grip is different: hold the plate with the thumbs up and fingers down.

Quick Tips

Explosive move with control challenges the core muscles and balance

2. Raise the plate over the head in an explosive motion, making sure to control the weight as it gets overhead. Hold for 1–2 seconds at the top, then slowly return to the starting position.

20. Hang Clean—Barbell

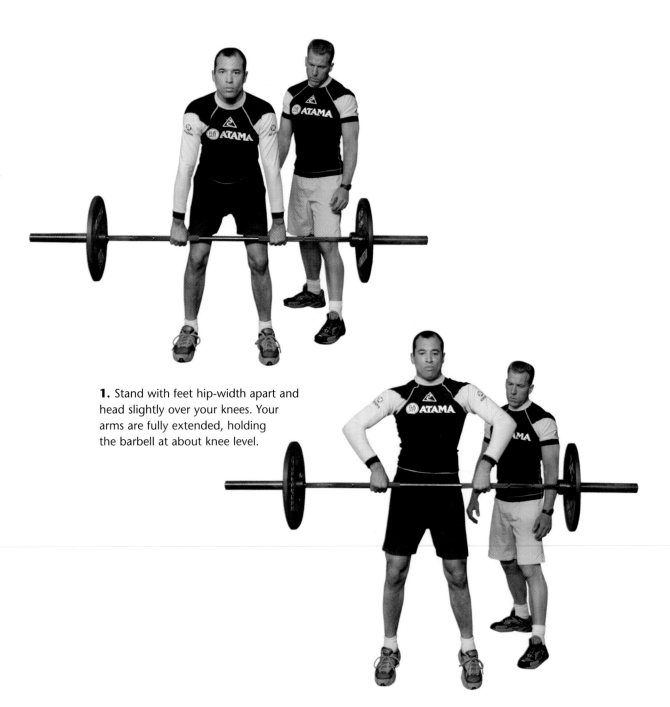

1. Stand with feet hip-width apart and head slightly over your knees. Your arms are fully extended, holding the barbell at about knee level.

2. In one explosive movement, shrug the shoulders up, pulling the barbell from thigh level to shoulder level. Pull the barbell as if you are jumping.

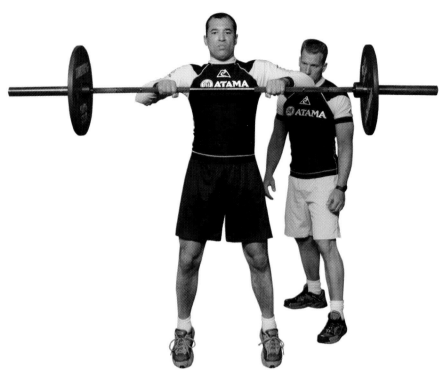

3. Keep the barbell level at all times.

Quick Tips
The barbell is the most difficult
 of the front raises
Great total body workout
Explosive movement
Can enhance your vertical jump
 as well

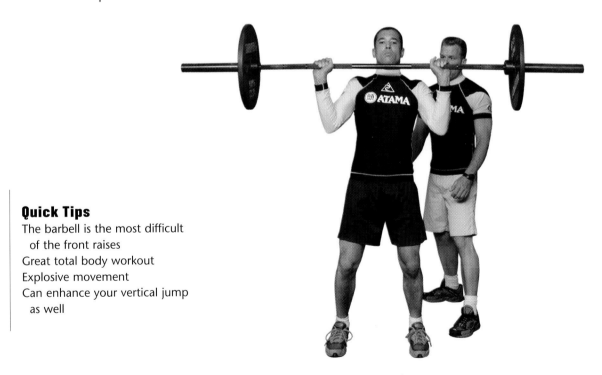

4. Catch the barbell by dropping the elbows and slightly bending the knees. Slowly return the barbell to the starting position.

21. Hang Clean—Dumbbell

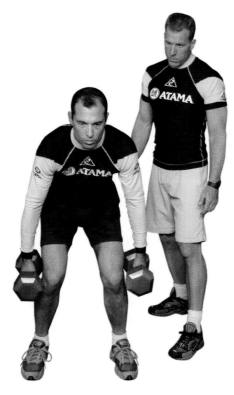

1. Stand with feet hip-width apart and head slightly over your knees. Your arms are fully extended, holding the dumbbells at about knee level.

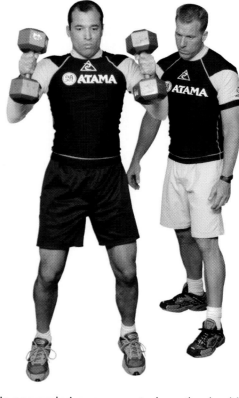

2. In one explosive movement, shrug the shoulders up, pulling the dumbbells from thigh level to shoulder level. Pull the dumbbells as if you are jumping.

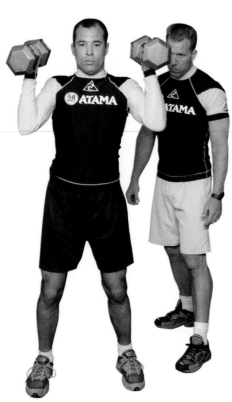

Quick Tips
Intermediate/Advanced
Great total body workout
Explosive movement
Can enhance your vertical jump as well

3. Catch the dumbbells by dropping the elbows and slightly bending the knees. Slowly return the dumbbells to the starting position.

22. High Pull—Dumbbell

1. Your stance should be wider than shoulder-width and your feet flat on the ground. Your knees are bent and your thighs should be parallel to the ground. Use a closed grip and position the dumbbell between your legs, slightly off the ground.

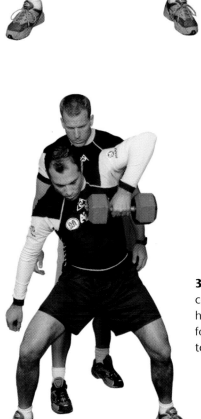

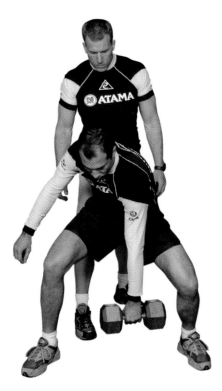

2. Once you are properly positioned on your starting point, quickly move the dumbbell up, using your hips and legs to propel the weight up in an explosive motion.

3. As the dumbbell passes your waist, use your arm to complete the upward movement. Your elbow should be higher than your shoulder. The upward momentum should force you up onto your toes. Control the dumbbell down to its starting point.

Quick Tips

Great for total body movement
Intermediate/Advanced
Your off hand can be resting on the knee or held away
  from the body
Great to develop coordination, control, and explosion

23. Hang Snatch—Dumbbell

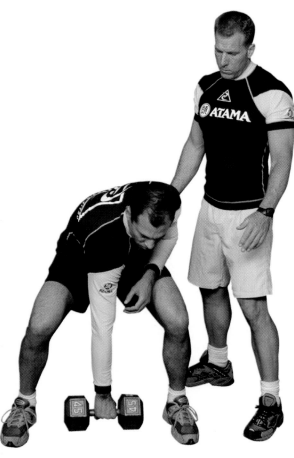

1. Stand with feet shoulder-width apart and slightly pointed outward. Your arm is completely extended, holding the dumbbell slightly off the ground between your feet. Position your head slightly over your knees.

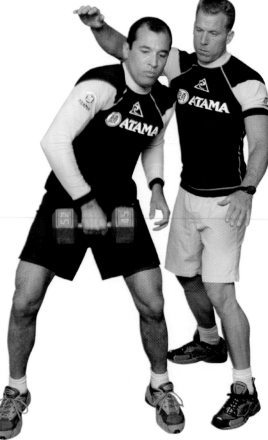

2. Begin your movement by straightening the knees and back. At this point your working arm is partially flexed and controlling the movement of the dumbbell. Keep the dumbbell close to your body.

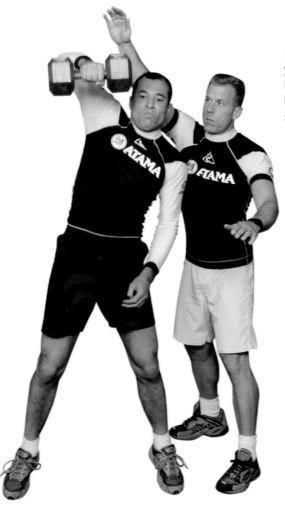

3. As the dumbbell travels past your shoulders, your working arm is in complete control of the dumbbell. Your elbow is high and you should be on the balls of your feet.

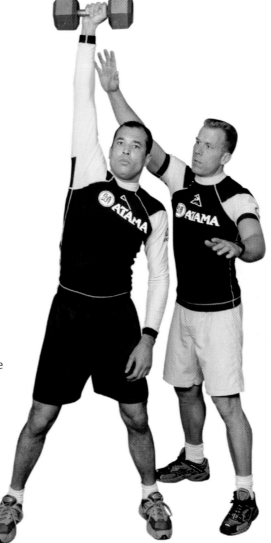

4. Control the movement of the dumbbell as your working arm becomes fully extended. Keep your base to provide the proper balance. Keep the dumbbell over your head.

Quick Tips
Intermediate/Advanced
Great total body workout
Explosive movement
Always use a spotter

24. Incline Press—Barbell

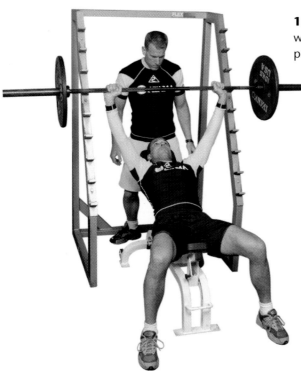

1. Start/finish: The overhand grip should be slightly wider than shoulder-width. The feet are flat and planted firmly on the ground.

2. Midpoint: The barbell is slowly lowered to the upper chest area until it touches. Make sure your feet remain flat on the ground.

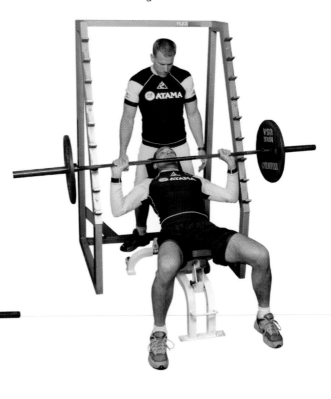

3. Detail: At this point, the barbell is pressed up in a straight line until the arms are completely extended back to the starting position.

Quick Tips

Incline at 45 degrees
Don't bounce the barbell off your chest
Always use a spotter

25. Incline Press—Dumbbell

1. Start/finish: Hold a dumbbell in each hand, palms facing forward. The dumbbells should be resting slightly above the chest, arms perpendicular to the floor.

Quick Tips

Rest the dumbbells on your
  thighs before you begin the lift
Always keep your buttocks on
  the bench
Use a 45-degree incline

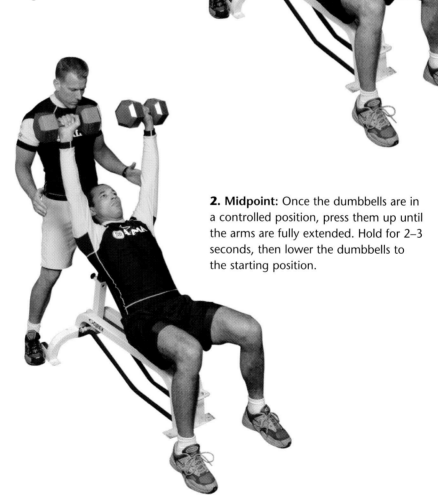

2. Midpoint: Once the dumbbells are in a controlled position, press them up until the arms are fully extended. Hold for 2–3 seconds, then lower the dumbbells to the starting position.

26. Incline Press—Narrow Grip Barbell

1. Start/finish: The overhand grip should be 6–8 inches apart. The bar rests on the upper chest area, elbows close to the body, feet flat on the ground.

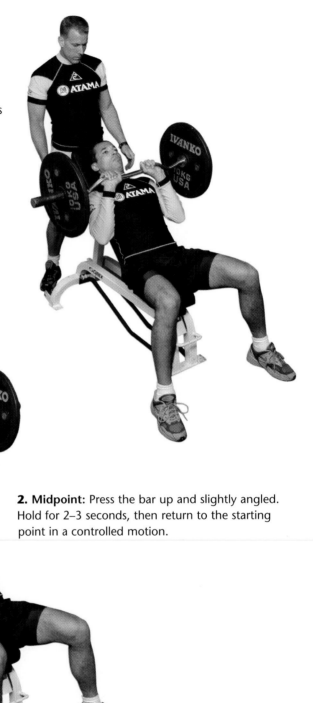

2. Midpoint: Press the bar up and slightly angled. Hold for 2–3 seconds, then return to the starting point in a controlled motion.

Quick Tips
You can use an EZ-curl bar or barbell if you like

27. Knee-Ups—Medicine Ball

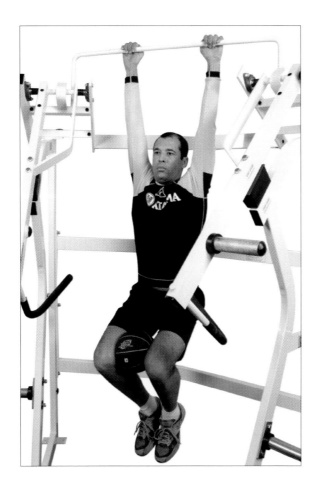

1. Grab a pull-up bar with your hands and trap a medicine ball between your legs.

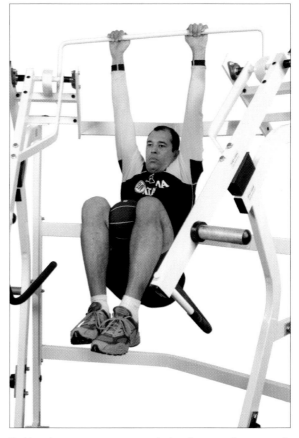

Quick Tips
Great for grip strength and endurance
You can use a towel or gi to add grip
 strength
Good for abs

2. Keeping your arms extended, raise your knees until the ball touches your chest. Lower and start over.

28. Lateral Raise—Dumbbell

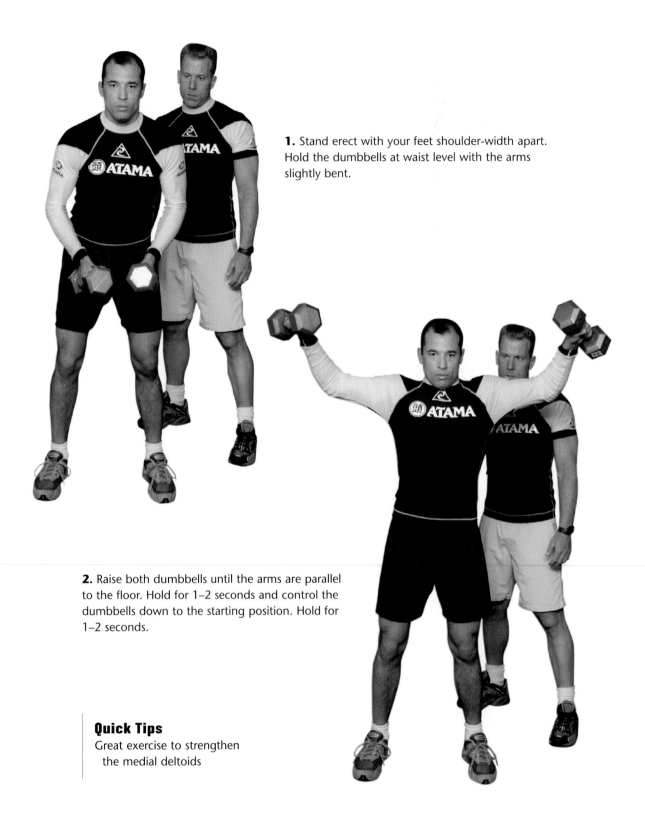

1. Stand erect with your feet shoulder-width apart. Hold the dumbbells at waist level with the arms slightly bent.

2. Raise both dumbbells until the arms are parallel to the floor. Hold for 1–2 seconds and control the dumbbells down to the starting position. Hold for 1–2 seconds.

Quick Tips
Great exercise to strengthen the medial deltoids

29. Lateral Raise—Dumbbell Seated

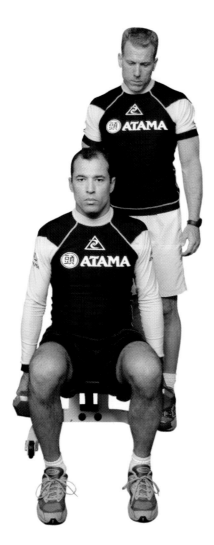

1. Hold the dumbbells at waist level with arms slightly bent. You will obtain greater isolation by sitting down, as you won't be able to use the legs to help the motion.

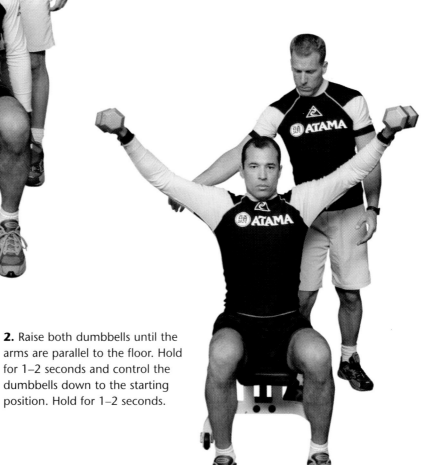

2. Raise both dumbbells until the arms are parallel to the floor. Hold for 1–2 seconds and control the dumbbells down to the starting position. Hold for 1–2 seconds.

Quick Tips
Intermediate/Advanced
Can be done isolateral as
   well for advanced

30. Lunges—Barbell

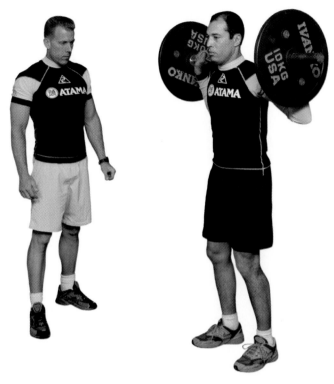

1. Stand erect with your feet shoulder-width apart. The barbell should be resting on your shoulders.

Quick Tips
Make sure the floor is level
Use collars on the barbell

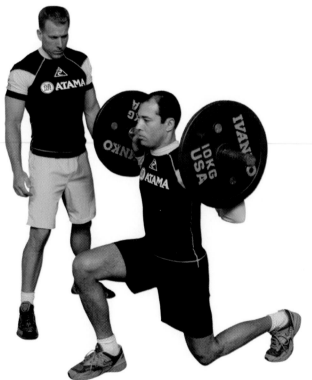

2. Slowly take a step forward with either leg, bending the knee of the lead leg. Lower your body until the back leg (knee) is slightly off the ground. Hold for 1–2 seconds, then push back with the lead leg, taking two or three small steps to return to the starting position.

31. Lunges—Dumbbell

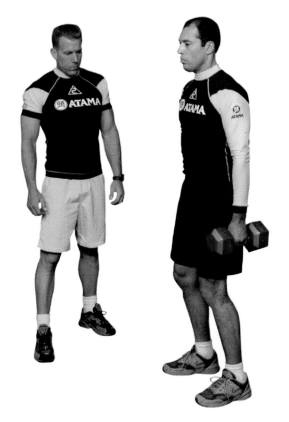

1. Stand erect with your feet shoulder-width apart. Hold the dumbbells at your sides.

Quick Tips
Make sure the floor is level
Keep the dumbbells from
  swinging

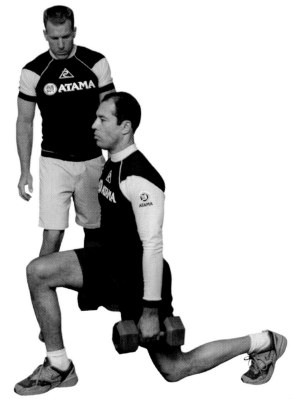

2. Slowly take a step forward with either leg, bending the knee of the lead leg. Lower your body until the back leg (knee) is slightly off the ground. Hold for 1–2 seconds, then push back with the lead leg, taking two or three small steps to return to the starting position.

32. Military Press—Barbell

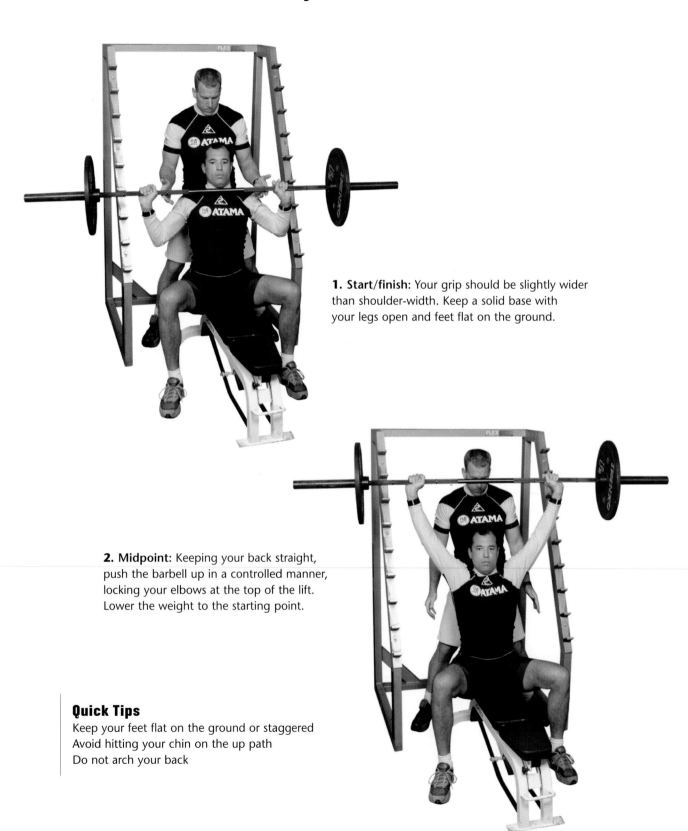

1. Start/finish: Your grip should be slightly wider than shoulder-width. Keep a solid base with your legs open and feet flat on the ground.

2. Midpoint: Keeping your back straight, push the barbell up in a controlled manner, locking your elbows at the top of the lift. Lower the weight to the starting point.

Quick Tips
Keep your feet flat on the ground or staggered
Avoid hitting your chin on the up path
Do not arch your back

33. Military Press—Dumbbell

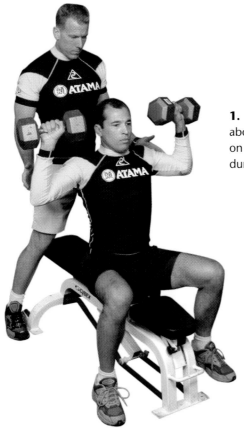

1. Start/finish: Hold the dumbbells slightly above the shoulders, keeping your feet flat on the floor and back straight. Balance the dumbbells before you begin the press.

2. Midpoint: Once the dumbbells are balanced, push them in a straight line above your head. When your arms are fully extended, hold for 2–3 seconds. Control the dumbbells down to the starting point.

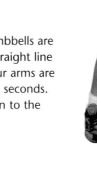

Quick Tips
Keep your back straight
Use a spotter

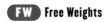

34. Military Press—Narrow Grip Barbell

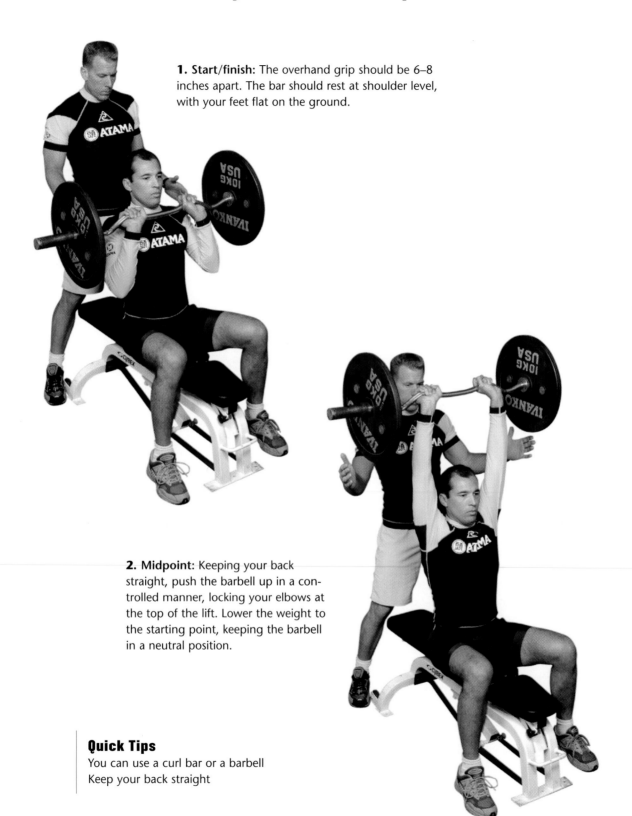

1. Start/finish: The overhand grip should be 6–8 inches apart. The bar should rest at shoulder level, with your feet flat on the ground.

2. Midpoint: Keeping your back straight, push the barbell up in a controlled manner, locking your elbows at the top of the lift. Lower the weight to the starting point, keeping the barbell in a neutral position.

Quick Tips

You can use a curl bar or a barbell
Keep your back straight

35. Pullovers—Barbell

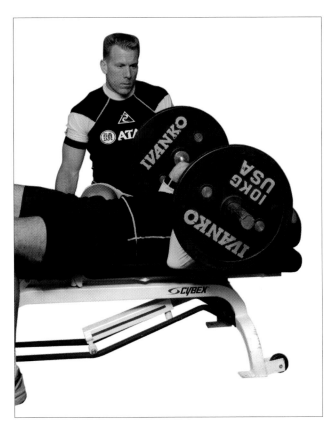

1. Position yourself flat on a bench with your feet firmly planted on the ground. Your grip should be narrow, 4–6 inches apart. Balance the barbell prior to starting the down movement, holding the barbell slightly off your chest.

Quick Tips
Can be combined with a press
To limit the range of motion of the pull, place the weight plates on the floor (lined up with the plates on the bar as a stopper)

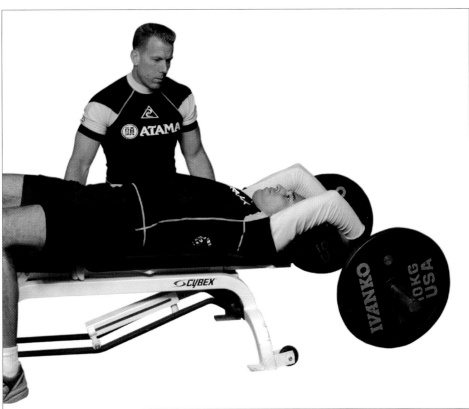

2. Slowly move the barbell over your head until it gently touches the floor. The barbell should always be about 6 inches above the face and head. After the barbell touches the floor, slowly pull it up to the starting position. Place weight plates on the ground to limit the range of motion.

36. Pullovers—Dumbbell

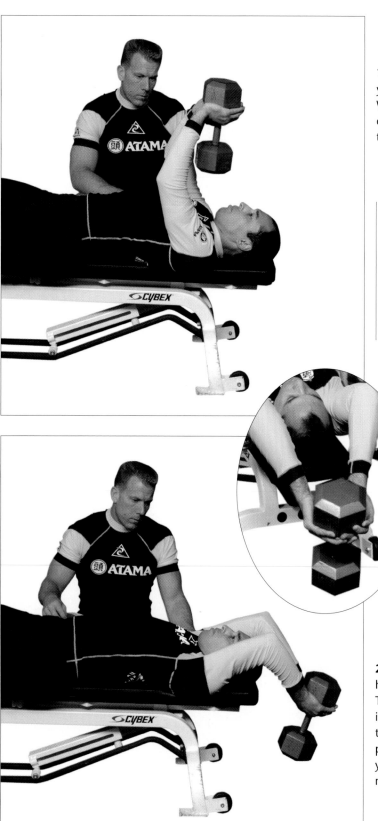

1. Position yourself flat on a bench with your feet firmly planted on the ground. With your arms extended, hold one end of the dumbbell in your fingers with a triangle grip.

Quick Tips

Use only fixed dumbbells
Great for shoulder flexibility
To limit the range of motion of the pull, place the weight plates on the floor (lined up with the dumbbell as a stopper)

Detail Once the dumbbell touches the floor, slowly move it back to the starting position. Keep the dumbbell away from your head.

2. Slowly move the dumbbell over your head until it gently touches the floor. The dumbbell should always be about 6 inches above the face and head. After the dumbbell touches the floor, slowly pull it up to the starting position. Keep your elbows bent on the down and up movements.

37. Pullovers—Towel

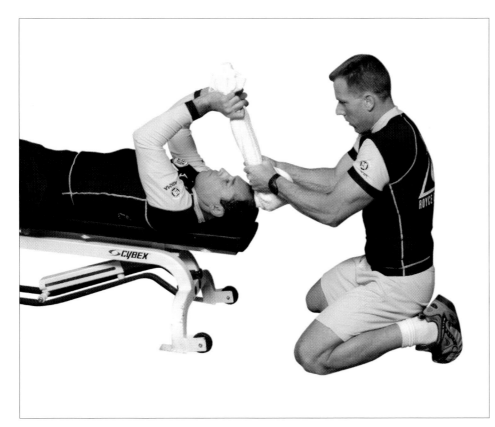

1. Position yourself flat on a bench with your feet firmly planted on the ground. With your arms extended, hold each end of the towel with your palms facing together. Keep a firm grip on the towel.

Quick Tips
Great for grip strength
Great for shoulder flexibility
Can be isometric with resistance at each end

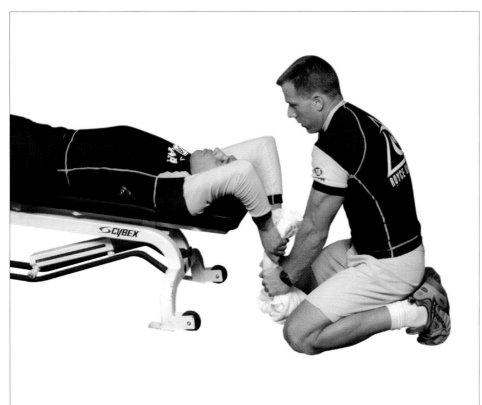

2. With resistance from your partner, slowly move the towel over your head until it touches the floor. Your wrists should always be 8–10 inches above your face and head. After the towel touches the floor, hold for 3–5 seconds. Slowly pull it up to the starting position. Your spotter can determine the range of motion and resistance.

38. Push Press—Barbell

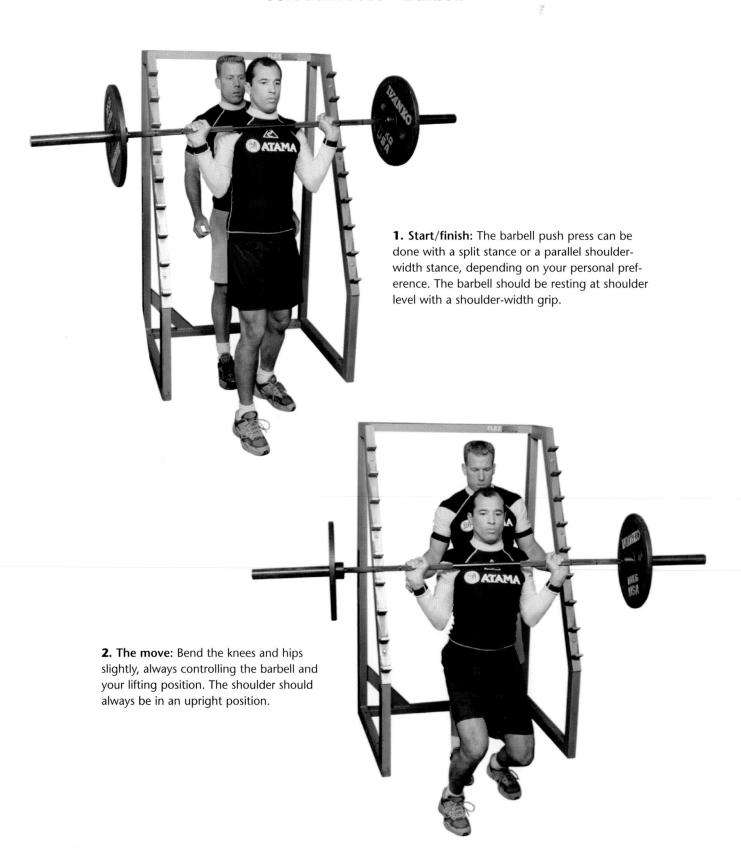

1. Start/finish: The barbell push press can be done with a split stance or a parallel shoulder-width stance, depending on your personal preference. The barbell should be resting at shoulder level with a shoulder-width grip.

2. The move: Bend the knees and hips slightly, always controlling the barbell and your lifting position. The shoulder should always be in an upright position.

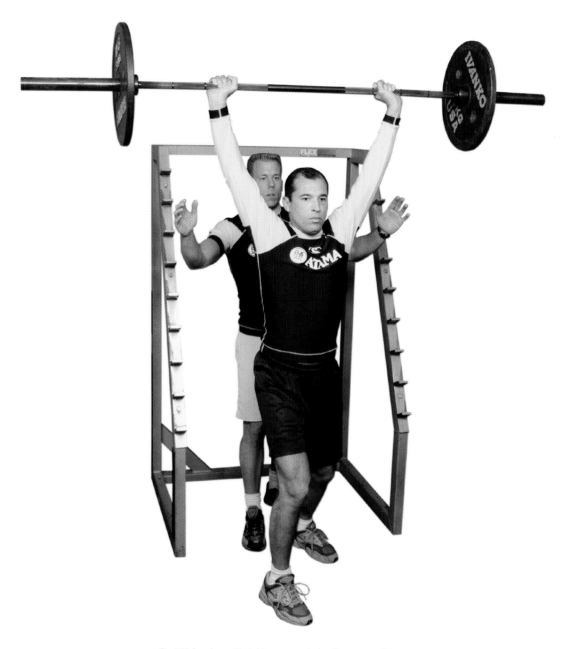

3. Midpoint: Quickly extend the knees and hips, pushing the barbell above your head. The force of the movement should come from the legs and hips.

Quick Tips

Do not let the bar roll forward
Find a balance point before you attempt the move
Use a spotter

39. Push Press—Dumbbell

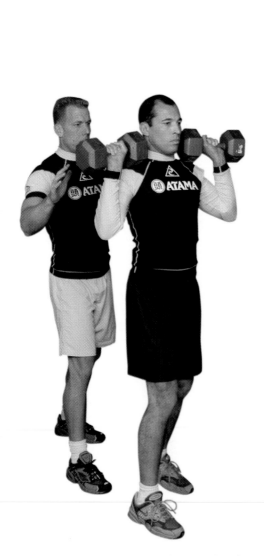 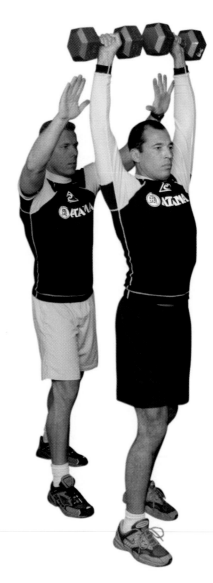

1. Start/finish: The push press can be completed with a split stance or a parallel shoulder-width stance. The dumbbells should be resting at shoulder level and shoulder width.

2. Midpoint: Once the dumbbells are stabilized, bend the knees and hips slightly and quickly extend them, pushing the dumbbells above your head. Hold the dumbbells in that position for 2–3 seconds. Lower the dumbbells in a controlled manner to the starting point.

Quick Tips

Alternate the lead foot from set to set
Find a comfortable stance before you begin
Use your legs to move the weight

40. Roll-Ups—Wrist

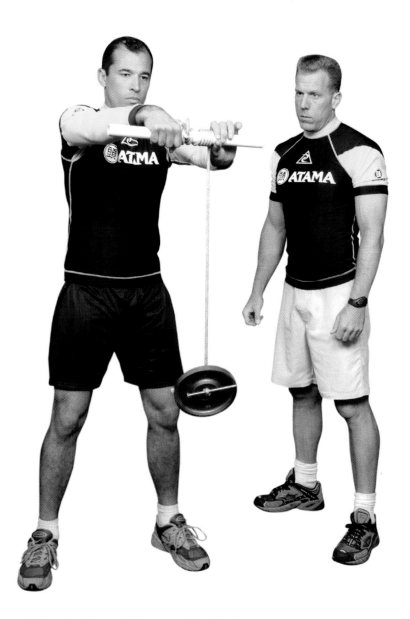

1. Your hands should be spaced 6–8 inches apart. Extend your arms outward at shoulder level. Using your hands, roll the weight up and then slowly roll it back to the starting position. The rope should be 3–4 feet long.

Quick Tips

Easy equipment to make
Great way to develop forearm strength

41. Row—Dumbbell

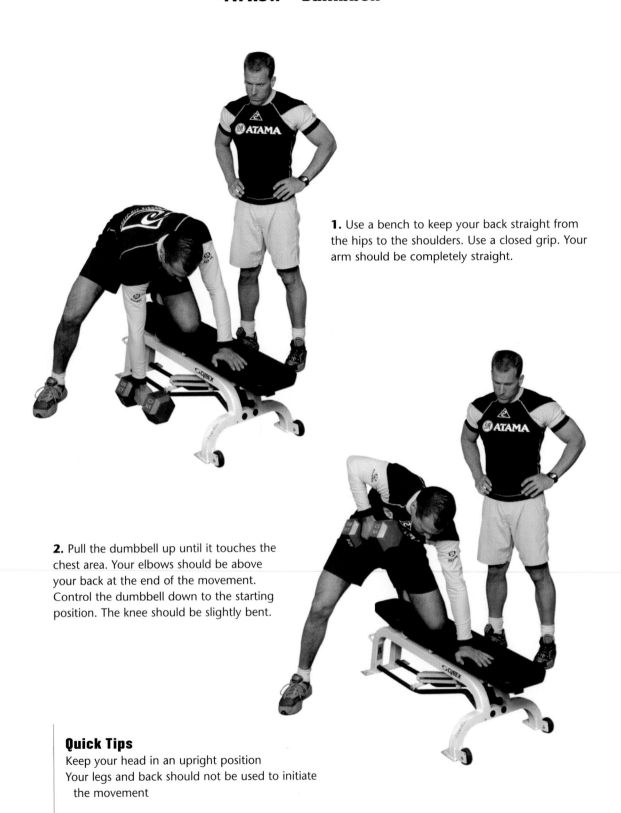

1. Use a bench to keep your back straight from the hips to the shoulders. Use a closed grip. Your arm should be completely straight.

2. Pull the dumbbell up until it touches the chest area. Your elbows should be above your back at the end of the movement. Control the dumbbell down to the starting position. The knee should be slightly bent.

Quick Tips

Keep your head in an upright position
Your legs and back should not be used to initiate
  the movement

42. Shoulder Shrugs—Barbell

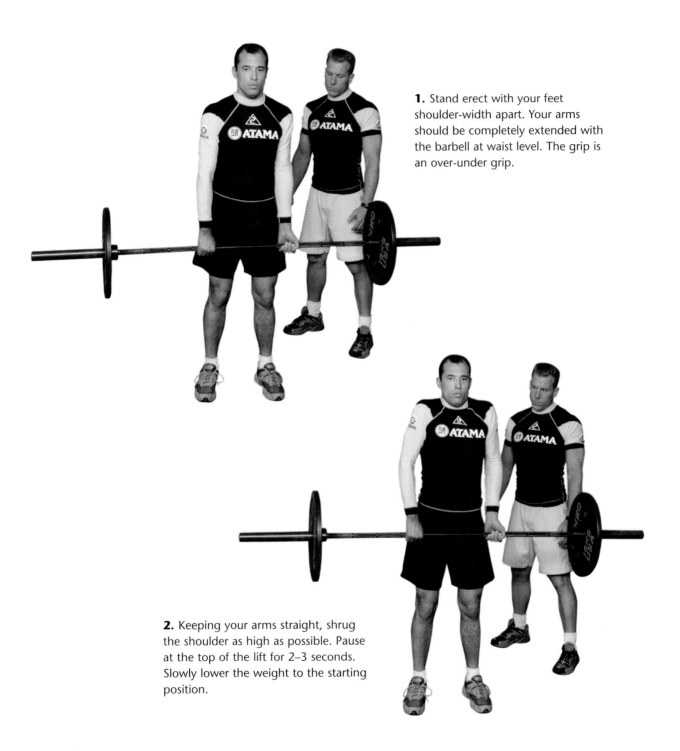

1. Stand erect with your feet shoulder-width apart. Your arms should be completely extended with the barbell at waist level. The grip is an over-under grip.

2. Keeping your arms straight, shrug the shoulder as high as possible. Pause at the top of the lift for 2–3 seconds. Slowly lower the weight to the starting position.

Quick Tips
Important to strengthen the trapezius and the neck

43. Shoulder Shrugs—Dumbbell

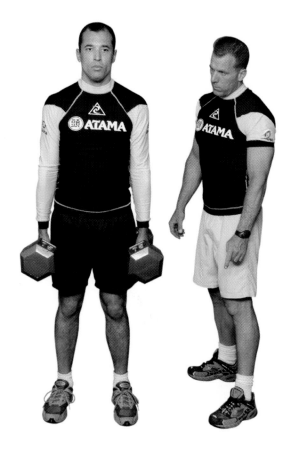

1. Stand erect with your feet shoulder-width apart. Your arms should be completely extended with the dumbbells at waist level. Dumbbells are a great way to assist with grip strength.

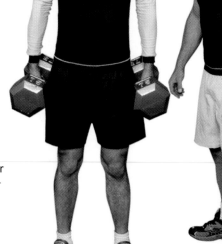

2. Keeping your arms straight, shrug the shoulder as high as possible. Pause at the top of the lift for 2–3 seconds. Slowly lower the dumbbells to the starting position.

Quick Tips

Great way to assist with grip strength
Important to strengthen the trapezius and the neck

43a: Hands-on Option

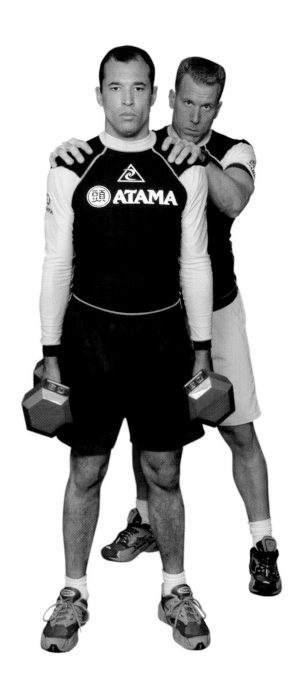

You can create more resistance by having a partner
exert pressure on your shoulder.

44. Squats—Barbell

1. Start/finish: Stand erect with your head in a neutral position. The arms are fully extended, holding the dumbbells at your sides. Your feet should be flat and shoulder-width apart.

2. Detail: Make sure you maintain the bar level and keep your back straight at all times, especially on the way up.

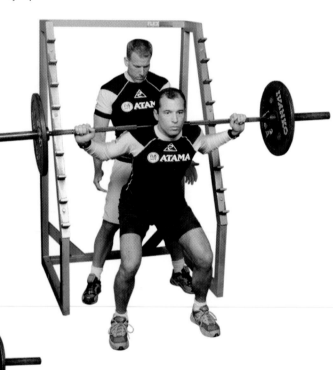

3. Midpoint: Bend the hips and knees until the thighs are parallel to the ground. Your shoulders should never extend over your knees. Hold for 1–2 seconds and return to the starting position.

Quick Tips
Intermediate/Advanced
Keep your back straight
Always use a spotter

45. Squats—Dumbbell

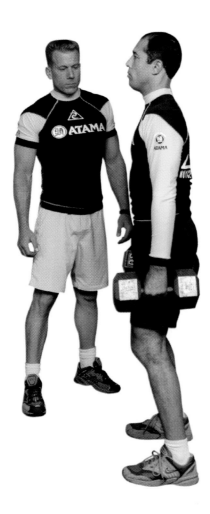

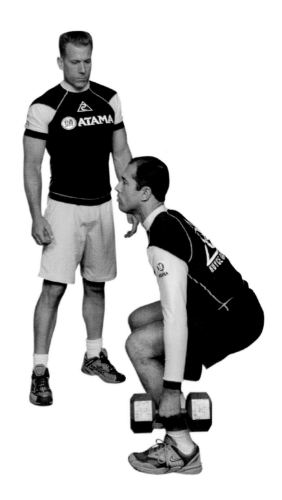

1. Start/finish: Stand erect with your head in a neutral position. The arms are fully extended, holding the dumbbells at your sides. Your feet should be flat and shoulder-width apart.

2. Midpoint: Bend the hips and knees until the thighs are parallel to the ground. Your shoulders should never extend over your knees. Hold for 1–2 seconds and return to the starting position.

Quick Tips
Good lift for beginners

46. Good Mornings

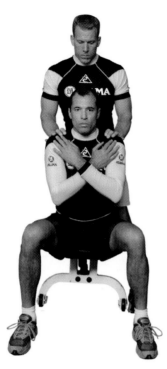

1. Sit on the end of a bench with your feet shoulder-width apart. Keep your back straight with your hands across your chest. Feet should be firmly planted on the ground.

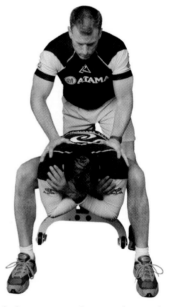

2. Slowly lower your chest and arms between your legs until you get a tolerable stretch.

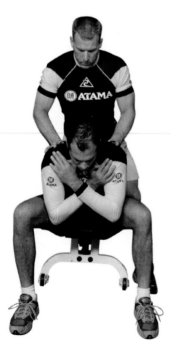

3. Once you have reached the down position, push back against the spotter's resistance. The primary push should come from the lower back region.

Quick Tips

In the absence of a spotter, hold a weight plate
Great lower-back stretch
Best with a spotter
Excellent abdominal workout

47. Reverse Hypers

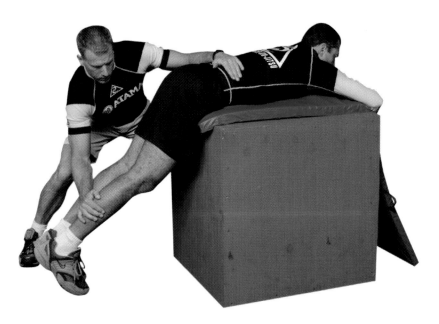

1. Lie face-down on a box with the edge of the box positioned at the hips. Grab the sides of the box for increased stability. The spotter applies resistance by holding the posterior side of your calves.

Quick Tips

Great exercise for lower back strength
Can also be done on a flat bench
Use an ankle weight for increased resistance
Can be done without resistance
Excellent abdominal workout

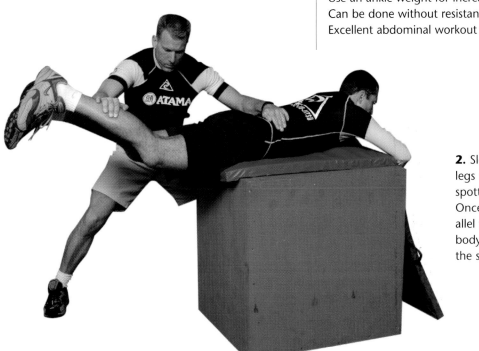

2. Slowly move your legs up against the spotter's resistance. Once your legs are parallel with your upper body, slowly return to the starting position.

48. Straight-Leg Dead Lifts—Barbell

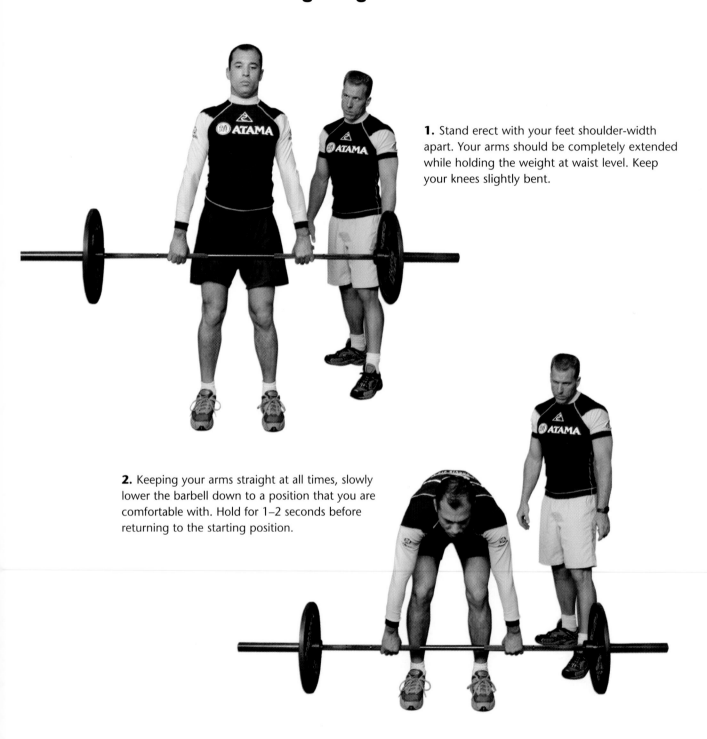

1. Stand erect with your feet shoulder-width apart. Your arms should be completely extended while holding the weight at waist level. Keep your knees slightly bent.

2. Keeping your arms straight at all times, slowly lower the barbell down to a position that you are comfortable with. Hold for 1–2 seconds before returning to the starting position.

Quick Tips

Advanced: Use a platform to increase range of motion

49. Straight-Leg Dead Lifts—Dumbbell

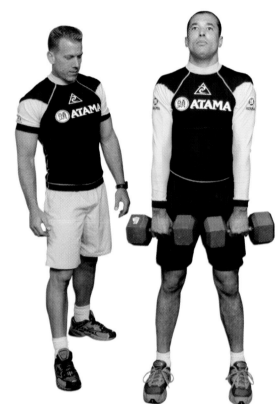

1. Stand erect with your feet shoulder-width apart. Your arms should be completely extended while holding the dumbbells at waist level. Keep your knees slightly bent.

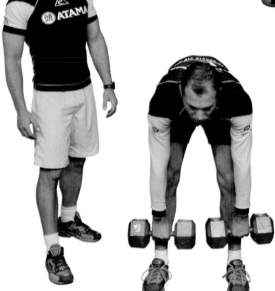

2. Keeping your arms straight at all times, slowly lower the dumbbells down to a position that you are comfortable with. Hold for 1–2 seconds before returning to the starting position.

Quick Tips

Advanced: Use a platform to increase the range of motion

50. Towel Grabs

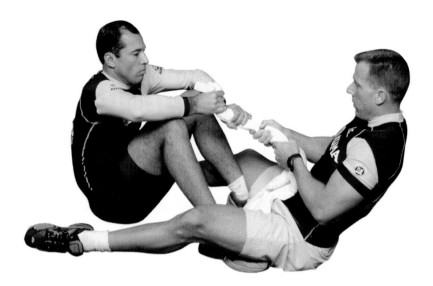

1. Sit with your feet hooked inside your spotter's thighs. Grab one end of the towel with your hands. The spotter grabs the other end to provide resistance.

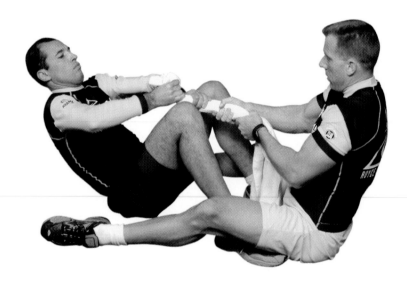

2. Start to lean back, pulling the towel and your spotter with you. Return to the start while resisting the spotter's pressure.

Quick Tips
Great for grip strength
Great for abs and back

51. Towel Pull-Ups

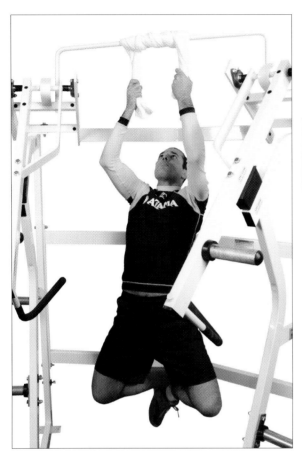

1. Wrap a thick towel around a chin-up bar and grab the ends with your hands.

Quick Tips

Great for grip strength and endurance

The thicker the towel, the harder the workout

You can use a gi instead of a towel and grab the collar to develop your choking or throwing grip

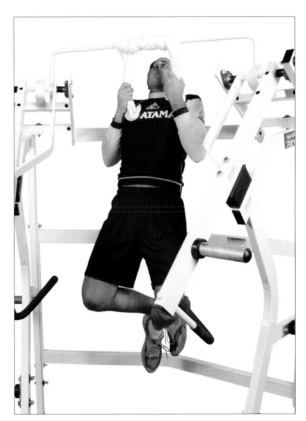

2. Pull yourself up, doing a regular pull-up until your elbows are next to your torso. Keep the elbows near your body.

52. Upright Row—Barbell

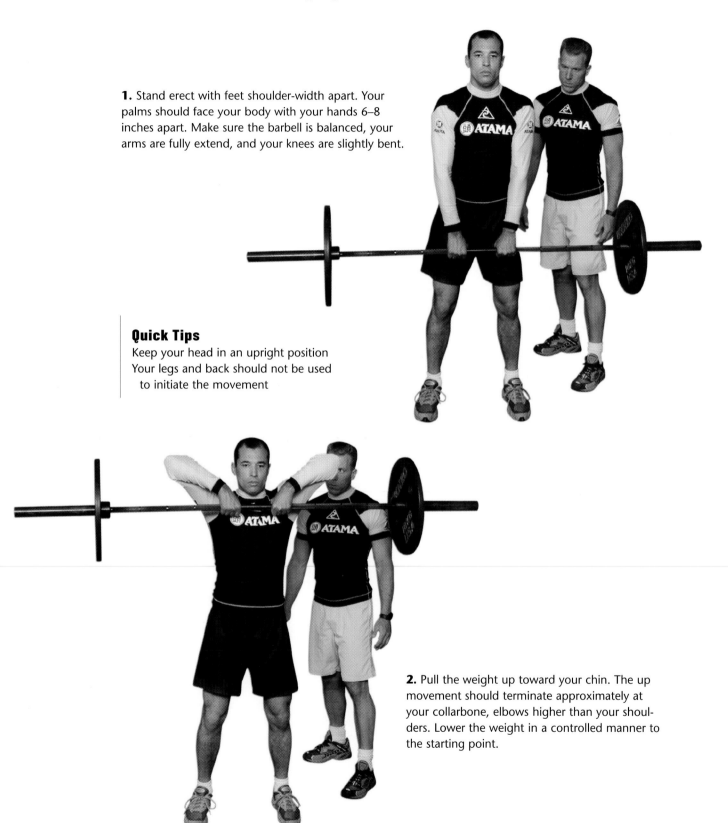

1. Stand erect with feet shoulder-width apart. Your palms should face your body with your hands 6–8 inches apart. Make sure the barbell is balanced, your arms are fully extend, and your knees are slightly bent.

Quick Tips
Keep your head in an upright position
Your legs and back should not be used
  to initiate the movement

2. Pull the weight up toward your chin. The up movement should terminate approximately at your collarbone, elbows higher than your shoulders. Lower the weight in a controlled manner to the starting point.

53. Upright Row—Dumbbell

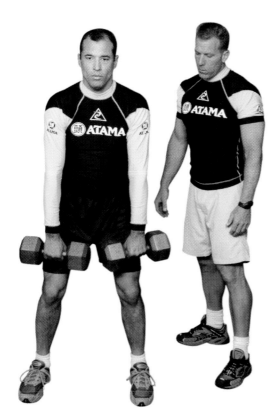

1. Stand erect with feet shoulder-width apart. Your palms should face your body. Make sure the dumbbells are balanced and your arms are fully extended.

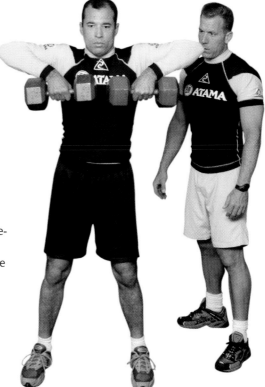

2. Pull the weight up toward your chin. The up movement should terminate approximately at your collarbone. Lower the weight in a controlled manner to the starting point, using only your shoulders to complete the movement.

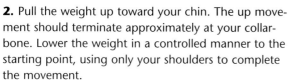

Quick Tips
Intermediate/Advanced
Great way to determine your dominant side

54. Upright Row—Plate

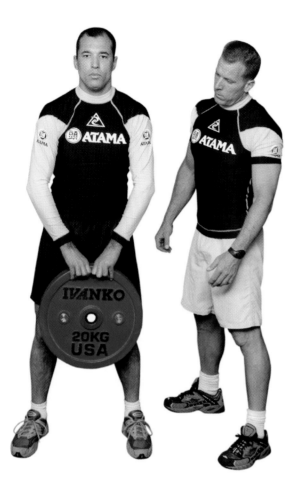

1. Stand erect with feet shoulder-width apart. Your palms should face your body and your hands should be 1–2 inches apart. Make sure the grip on the plate is solid and the hands are close together.

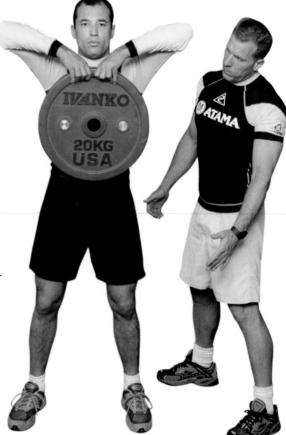

2. Pull the weight up toward your chin. The up movement should terminate approximately at your collarbone, elbows higher than your shoulders. Lower the weight in a controlled manner to the starting point.

Quick Tips
Great lift for beginners
Great way to develop finger and grip strength

55. Upright Row—Towel

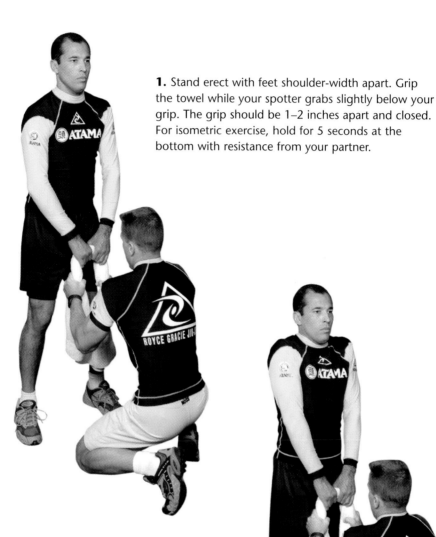

1. Stand erect with feet shoulder-width apart. Grip the towel while your spotter grabs slightly below your grip. The grip should be 1–2 inches apart and closed. For isometric exercise, hold for 5 seconds at the bottom with resistance from your partner.

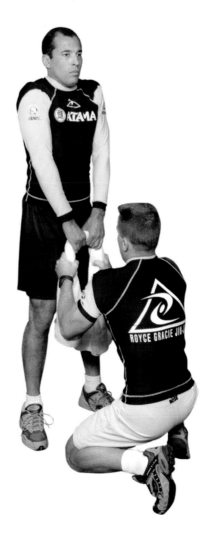

2. Pull the towel up toward your chin. The up movement should terminate slightly above chest level with constant resistance from your partner. For isometric exercise, hold for 5 seconds at the top with resistance from your partner.

Quick Tips
Great for grip strength improvement
Can be isometric or not (with or without the 5-second hold)

56. Rice Grabs

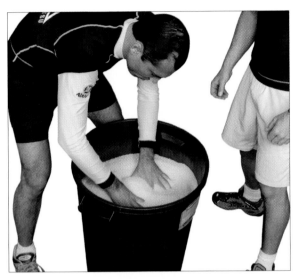

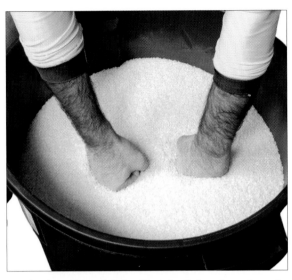

1. Stationary Open Grip: Place both hands on top of the rice. Fingers should be wide apart. Once your hands are set, quickly close and open your hands, squeezing the rice.

2. Digging Closed Grip: Place both hands on top of the rice with a closed grip (making a fist). Push and rotate your hands down until the rice is just below your elbows and return to the start.

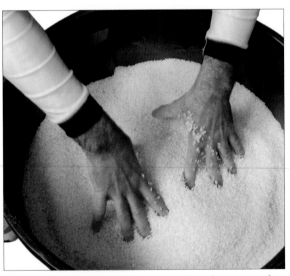

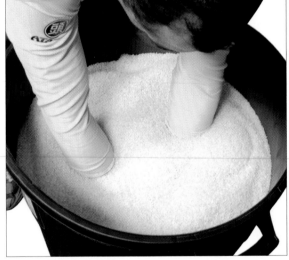

3. Digging Open Grip: Place both hands on top of the rice with fingers wide apart.

4. Quickly open and close your hands while pushing down until the rice is just below your elbows. Do the same thing with one hand only.

Quick Tips
Great for grip strength and endurance

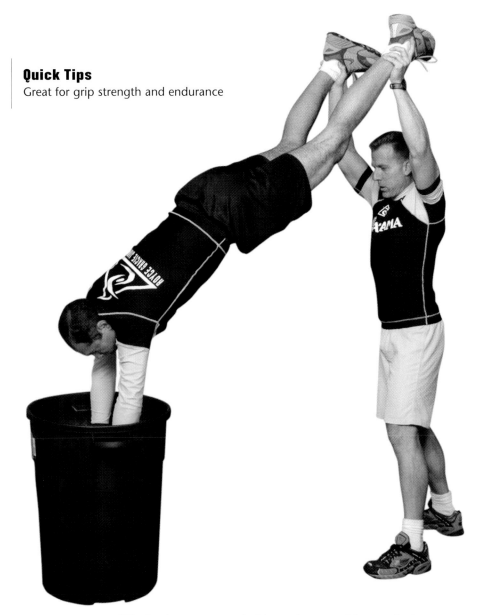

5. For greater difficulty, have a spotter hold your legs up while you do these same exercises.

ISOLATERALS **ISO**

57. Bench Press—Isolateral

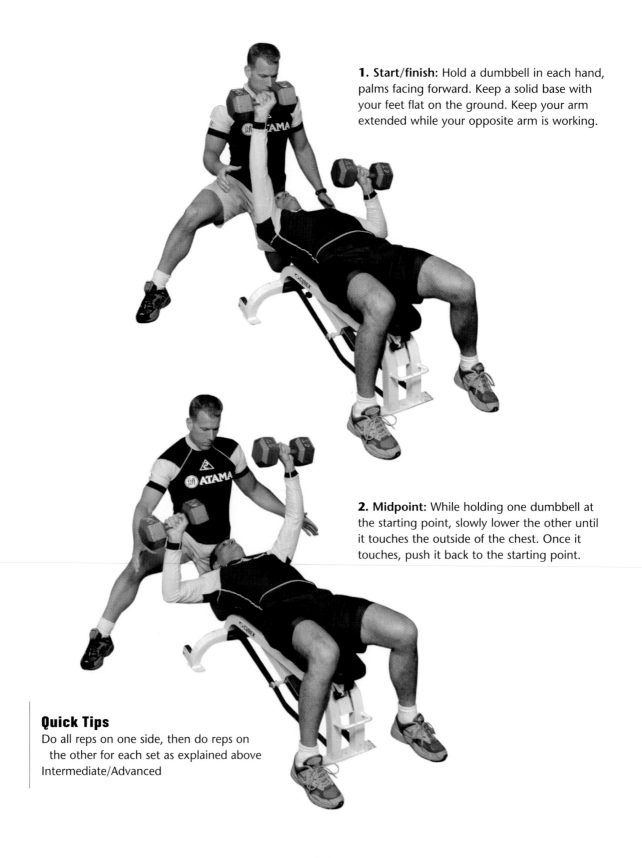

1. Start/finish: Hold a dumbbell in each hand, palms facing forward. Keep a solid base with your feet flat on the ground. Keep your arm extended while your opposite arm is working.

2. Midpoint: While holding one dumbbell at the starting point, slowly lower the other until it touches the outside of the chest. Once it touches, push it back to the starting point.

Quick Tips

Do all reps on one side, then do reps on the other for each set as explained above
Intermediate/Advanced

58. Front Raise—Isolateral

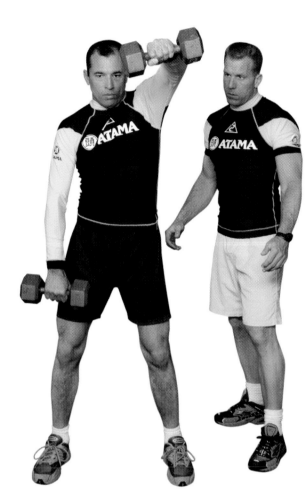

1. Stand erect with feet approximately shoulder-width apart, holding a dumbbell in each hand. Work one side at a time.

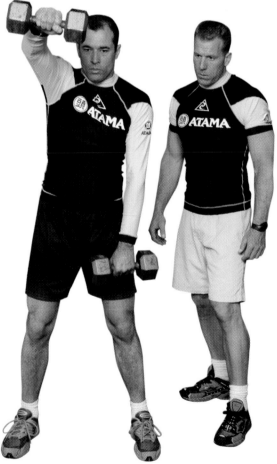

2. Raise the dumbbell to eye level. Hold for 1–2 seconds at the top, then slowly return to the starting position.

Quick Tips
Great exercise to strengthen the anterior deltoid

59. Incline Press—Isolateral

1. Start/finish: Hold a dumbbell in each hand, palms facing forward. Keep a solid base with your feet flat on the ground. Keep your arm extended while the opposite arm is working.

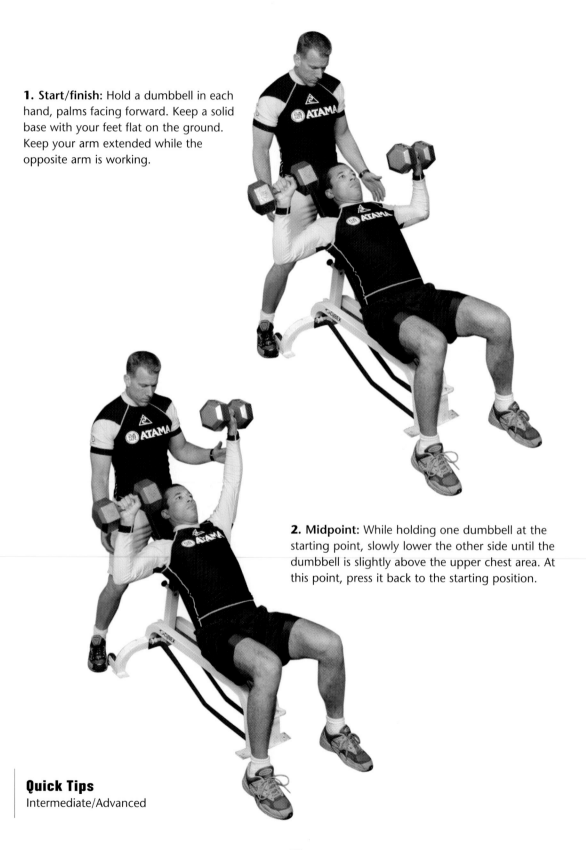

2. Midpoint: While holding one dumbbell at the starting point, slowly lower the other side until the dumbbell is slightly above the upper chest area. At this point, press it back to the starting position.

Quick Tips
Intermediate/Advanced

60. Lateral Raise—Isolateral

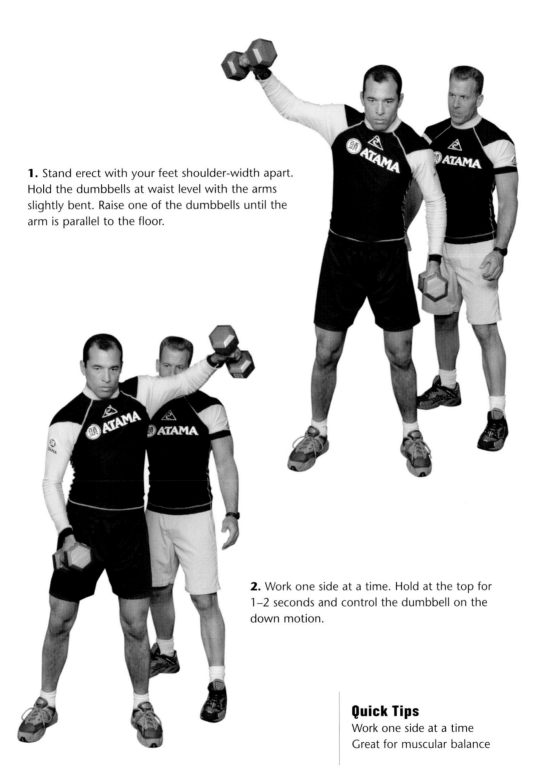

1. Stand erect with your feet shoulder-width apart. Hold the dumbbells at waist level with the arms slightly bent. Raise one of the dumbbells until the arm is parallel to the floor.

2. Work one side at a time. Hold at the top for 1–2 seconds and control the dumbbell on the down motion.

Quick Tips

Work one side at a time
Great for muscular balance

61. Military Press—Isolateral

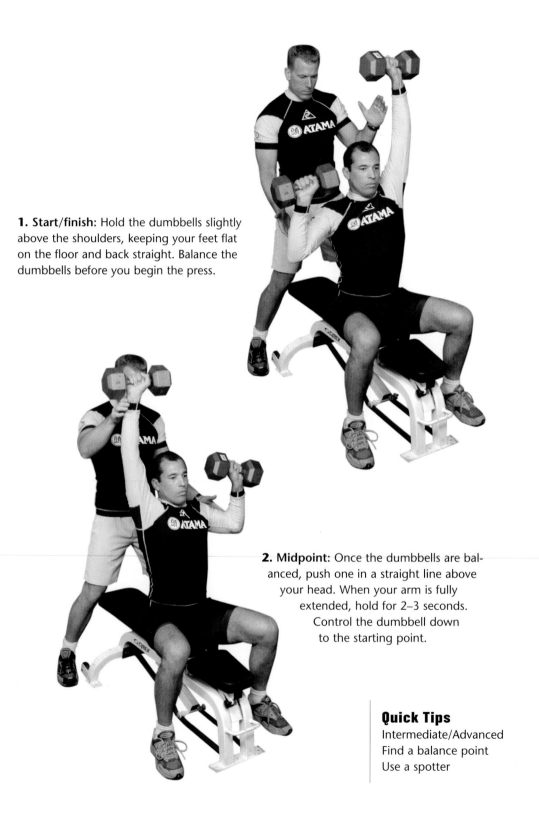

1. Start/finish: Hold the dumbbells slightly above the shoulders, keeping your feet flat on the floor and back straight. Balance the dumbbells before you begin the press.

2. Midpoint: Once the dumbbells are balanced, push one in a straight line above your head. When your arm is fully extended, hold for 2–3 seconds. Control the dumbbell down to the starting point.

Quick Tips
Intermediate/Advanced
Find a balance point
Use a spotter

62. Push Press—Isolateral

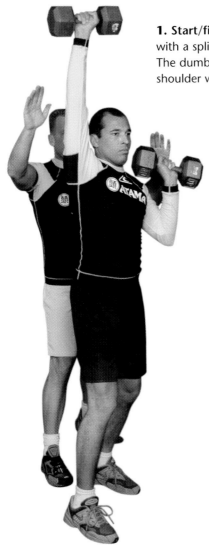

1. Start/finish: The push press can be completed with a split stance or a parallel shoulder-width stance. The dumbbells should be resting at shoulder level and shoulder width.

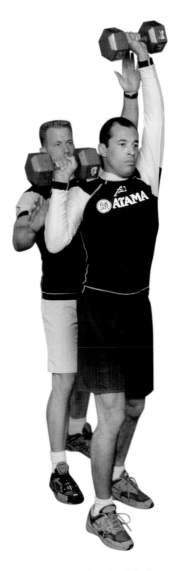

Quick Tips
Intermediate/Advanced
Alternate the lead foot with each set
Know your dominant side so you work the
   opposite side to balance your muscles
Use a spotter

2. Midpoint: Once the dumbbells are stabilized, bend the knees and hips slightly and quickly extend one arm, pushing one dumbbell above your head while holding the other at chest level. Hold the dumbbell in that position for 2–3 seconds. Lower the dumbbell in a controlled manner to the starting point. After one set, switch and do the other side.

63. Upright Row—Isolateral

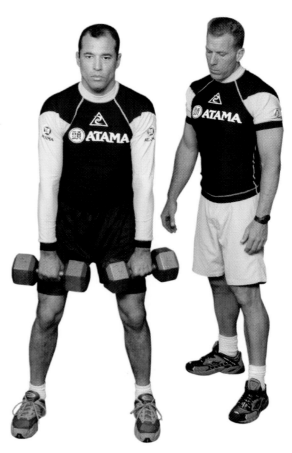

1. Stand erect with feet shoulder-width apart. Your hands should be 6–8 inches apart. Make sure the dumbbells are balanced and your arms are fully extended. Pull the weight up towards your chin.

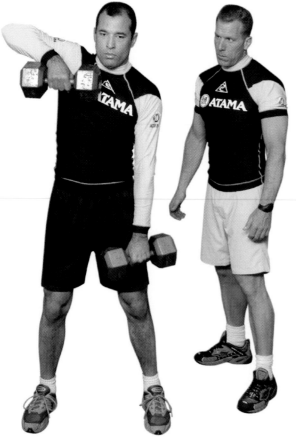

2. Work one side at a time. The up movement should terminate approximately at your collarbone. Lower the weight in a controlled manner to the starting point.

Quick Tips
Can be done by beginners as well as advanced lifters

Great way to develop strength on your nondominant side

64. Machine Cross

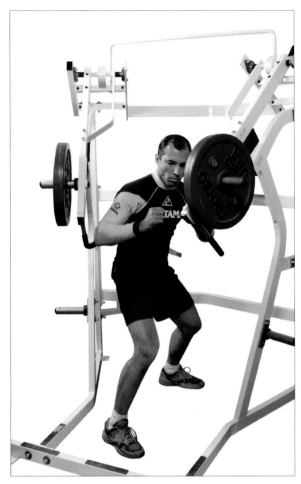

1. Stand in a sideways stance with your back arm pushing against the grip.

Quick Tips
Use a lighter weight at first

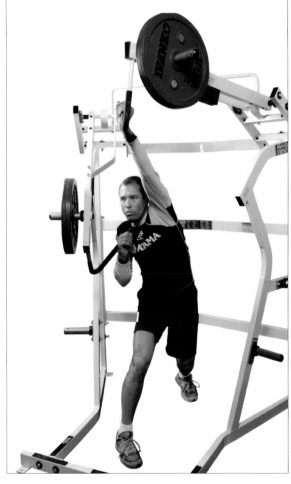

2. Pushing off your rear leg, pivot on the ball of your foot and push the handle forward as if you were delivering a punch. Make sure you drive the punch all the way through.

65. Machine Uppercut

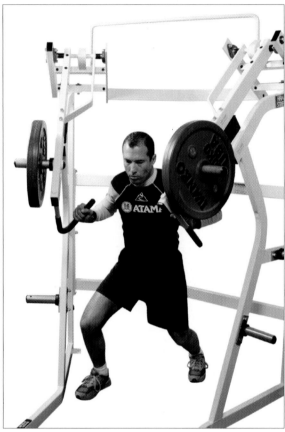

1. Stand in a split stance with your arms pushing against the grips.

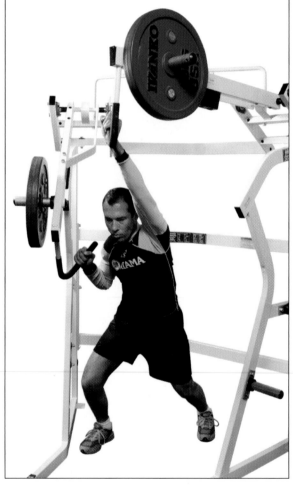

2. Pushing off your rear leg, drive the handle forward as if you were delivering a punch. Make sure you drive the punch all the way through.

Quick Tips
Use a lighter weight at first
Switch feet and work both sides
  equally

PLYOMETRICS **PL**

66. Box Jumps

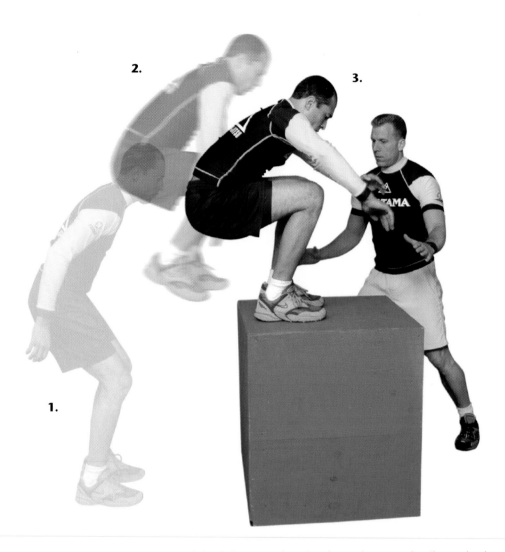

1. Stand in front of the box with both feet together. Bend your knees and coil your body.

2. Pushing off your legs, do an explosive jump up to the top of the box.

3. Land with both feet at the same time close together. Jump back down to the start position.

Quick Tips

Make sure the box is steady
Start with a box that is not too high so you can accomplish the jump
Be careful not to miss the landing
Land on the balls of your feet
Bend at the knees when landing
Intermediate (use a knee-high box) /Advanced (use a higher box)

67. Box Jumps—One Leg

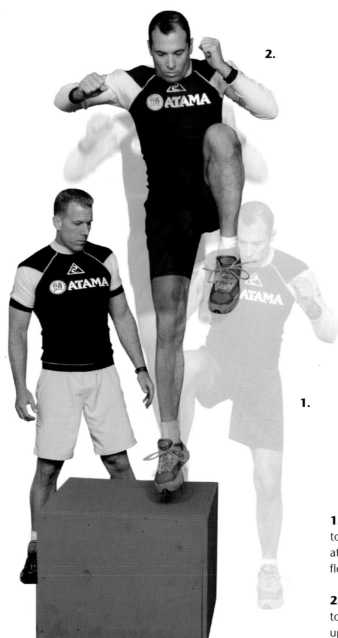

2.

1.

1. Stand with one foot firmly placed on top of the box. Hands should be held at shoulder level. Thigh is parallel to the floor.

2. With one quick motion, extend the top leg while bringing the opposite leg up to your chest. The movement should be a quick jump.

3. Return to the starting position and repeat the motion. Make sure you repeat the exercise with the other leg and work both sides equally.

Quick Tips
Great exercise to develop leg strength

68. Lateral Jumps

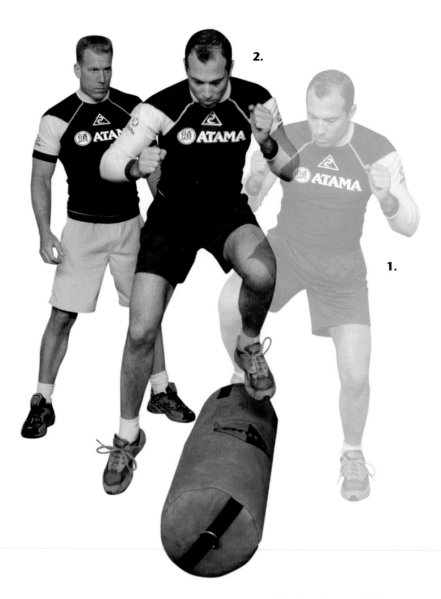

2.

1.

1. Begin the exercise with one foot on the bag and the leg bent, with the thigh parallel to the floor. Your foot should be placed firmly on the bag. Hands should be shoulder level.

2. With a quick motion, extend the bent leg and jump to the other side of the bag. Quickly repeat the motion to the opposite side.

Quick Tips

Can be used as a warm-up
Land on the balls of your feet
Bend at the knees when landing
Good speed drill for quick feet
Good plyometric and endurance exercise

69. Lateral Jumps—Long Way

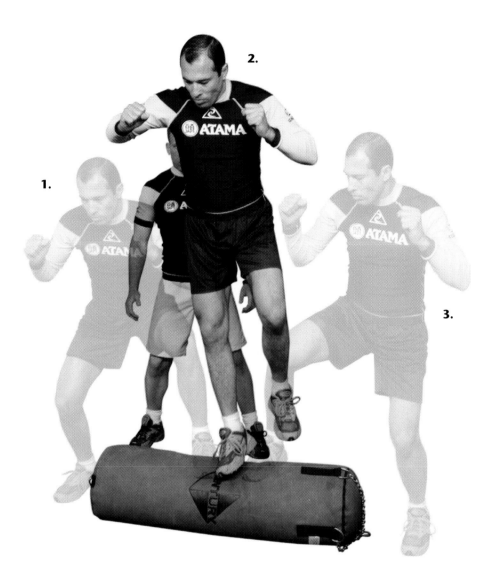

1. Begin the exercise with one foot near the middle of the bag. Your foot should be placed firmly on the bag. Hands should be shoulder level. The opposite or down leg should be slightly bent.

2. With a quick motion, extend the top leg while pushing off with the opposite leg.

3. Make sure your lag foot lands toward the center of the bag. Once you land, repeat the motion and work both sides equally.

Quick Tips
Intermediate/Advanced
Great way to develop lateral movement

70. Lateral Jumps—Short Way

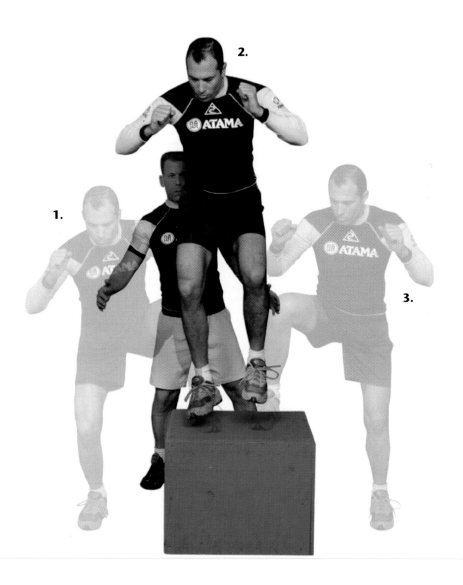

1. Stand with one foot firmly placed on the top of the box. Hands should be held at shoulder level. The opposite or down leg should be slightly bent.

2. With one explosive motion, extend the top leg while pushing off with the opposite leg. Use a quick and powerful push!

3. Make sure your lag foot lands toward the center of the box. Once you land, repeat the motion and work both sides equally.

Quick Tips
Intermediate/Advanced
Great way to develop lateral movement

71. Medicine Ball Ground Work—One Hand

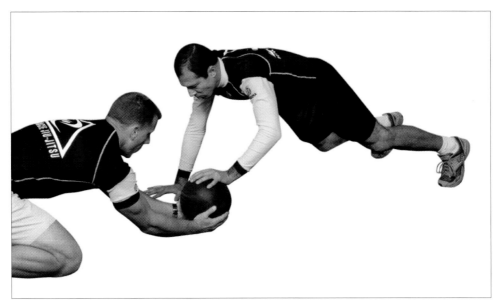

1. Start by placing one hand on the ball and the other on the ground. Your legs are wide apart and your arms slightly bent. The goal is to move your hands back and forth over the ball.

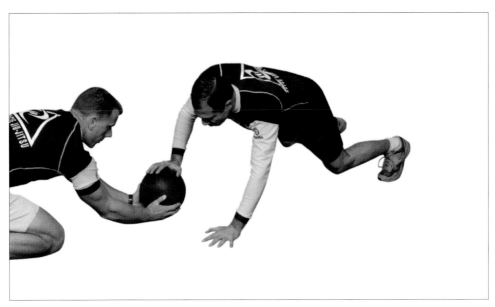

2. Quickly move one hand off the ball as the other hand comes on to the ball. Move your feet in the same direction as your hands. Use quick lateral movement over the ball.

Quick Tips
Great for upper body endurance
Good upper-body plyometric exercise
Great for lateral movement and eye-body coordination
Always use a spotter

72. Medicine Ball Ground Work—Two Hands

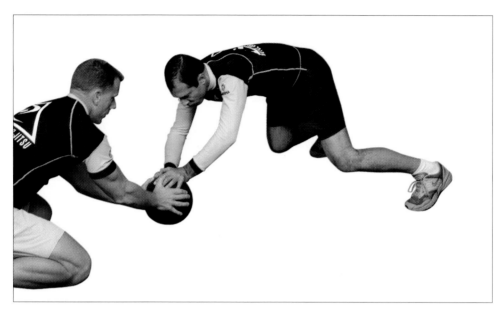

1. Start by placing both hands firmly on the top of the ball. Your legs are wide apart and your arms slightly bent. Your spotter must hold the ball firmly.

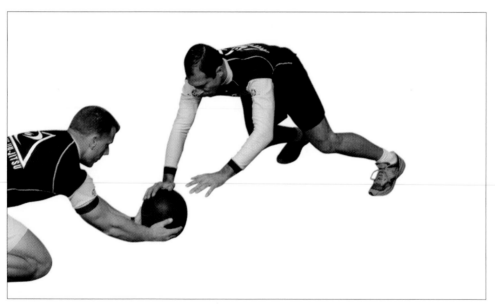

2. Quickly move your hands laterally off the ball until both hands are on the ground. As soon as the second hand touches the ground, place your hand back on the ball, moving in the opposite direction.

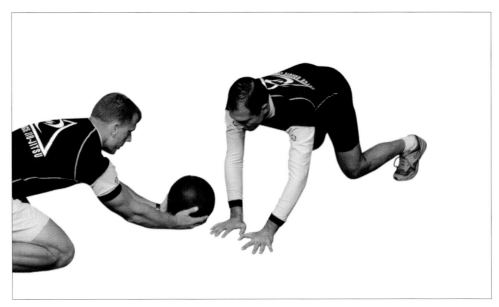

3. Move that hand onto the ground as the second hand moves onto the ball. It is important to move your feet slightly in the same direction as your hands.

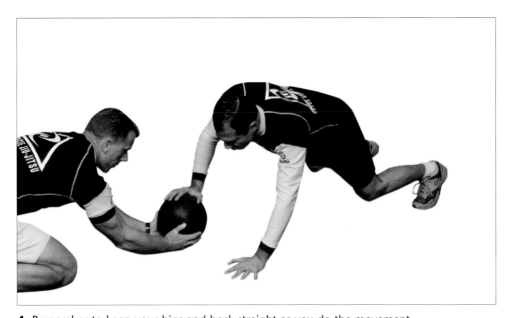

4. Remember to keep your hips and back straight as you do the movement.

Quick Tips

Great for upper body strength and endurance

Good upper-body plyometric exercise

Great for lateral movement and eye-body coordination

Intermediate/Advanced

Always use a spotter

Go to both sides

73. Medicine Ball Toss—Flat Bench

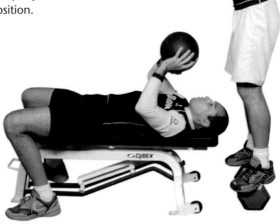

1. Position yourself directly underneath your spotter. Your feet should be flat on the ground with your back slightly arched. Your hands should be in a "V" position with the medicine ball resting equally on both hands. Always start in the down position.

2. Push the medicine ball up with one explosive motion. As the ball moves up toward the spotter, keep your hands in a ready position to receive the ball. The spotter does not catch the ball; he controls the flight so that the lifter can catch the ball and repeat the process. The spotter can stand on a box for increased distance.

Quick Tips
Great for upper-body endurance
Must have a spotter

74. Medicine Ball Walk/Hold/Balance

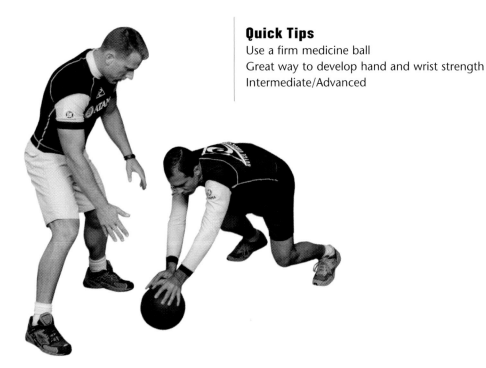

Quick Tips
Use a firm medicine ball
Great way to develop hand and wrist strength
Intermediate/Advanced

1. Walk: Position your hands firmly on top of the ball with your feet shoulder-width apart. Slowly push the ball forward, using your hands to move the ball. Keep your hands on top of the ball throughout the entire movement.

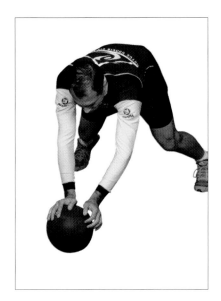

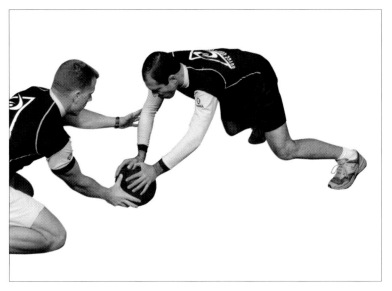

2. Hold: Position your hands on top of the ball. Your feet should be in a wide stance to help your balance.

3. Balance: The spotter quickly rotates the medicine ball back and forth. As the medicine ball rotates, reposition your hands to maintain your balance.

75. Push-Ups—Plyometric

1. Stack two sets of plates approximately shoulder width apart on the mat. Get in a push-up stance with your hands just inside the plates, touching the ground. Bend your arms and bring your chest close to the ground.

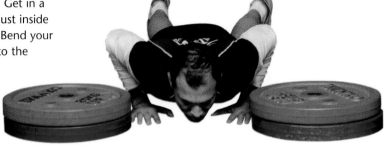

2. Pushing off your arms, explode upwards and touch the top of the plates quickly.

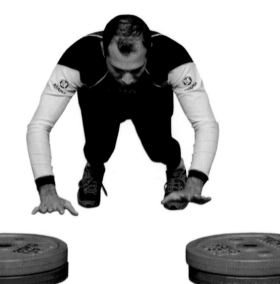

3. Land with your hands inside the plates, bring your chest to the ground, and quickly repeat the motion.

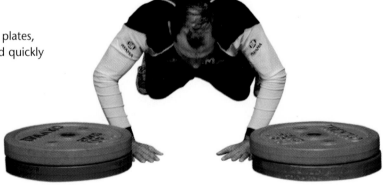

Quick Tips
Great endurance exercise
Intermediate/Advanced
Stack more plates for greater challenge

76. Step-Ups—Body Weight

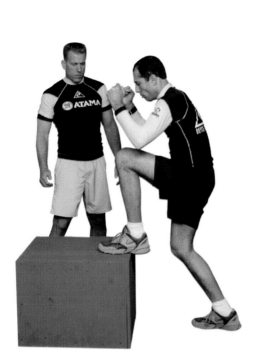

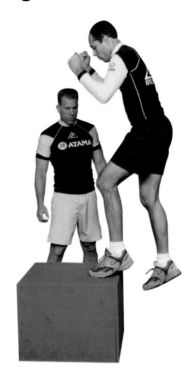

1. Stand with one foot firmly placed on top of the box. Hands should be held at shoulder level. Thigh is parallel to the floor, the opposite or down leg slightly bent.

2. With one quick and powerful motion, extend the top leg while pushing off the down leg. Switch your feet in the air as you go down.

Quick Tips
Intermediate/Advanced
Can use a flat bench
  instead of a box

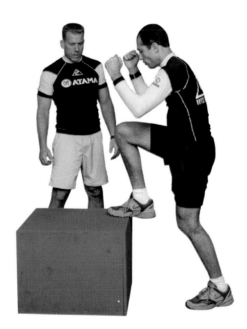

3. Quickly repeat the exercise once the opposite leg touches the box.

POWER SERIES PS

77. Cones Workout

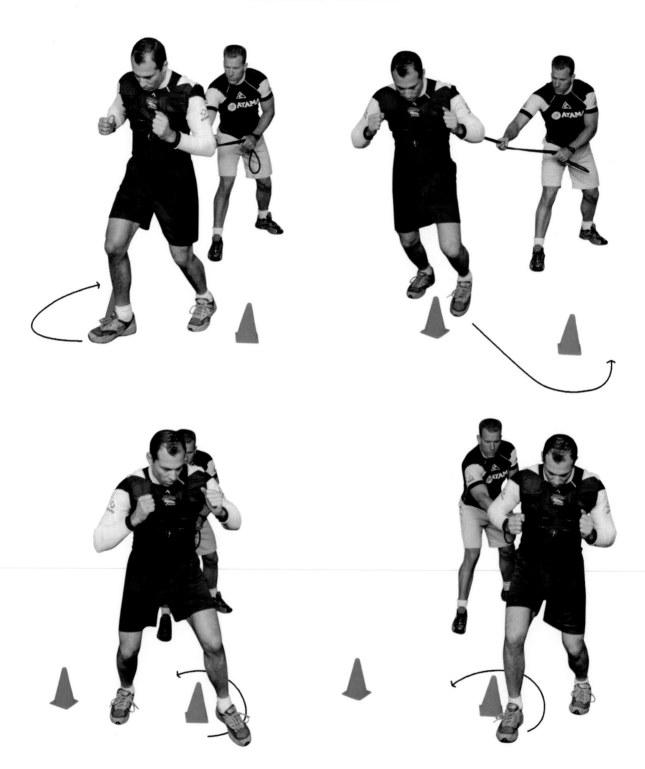

1. Figure 8s—Standing
Standing Circle around the cones, doing figure-8s and shuffling your feet.

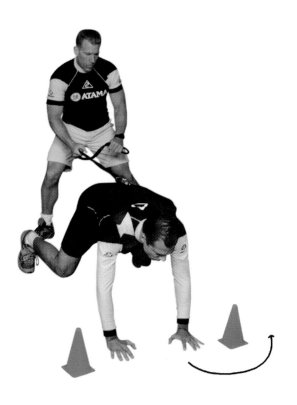

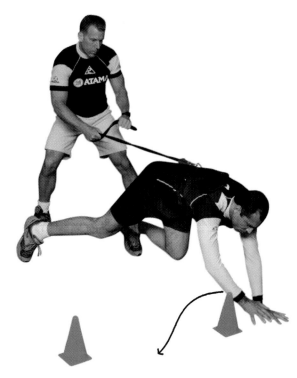

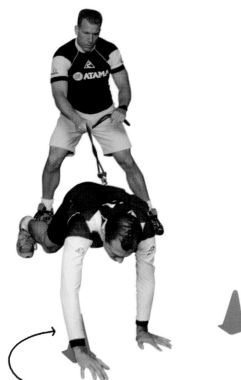

2. Figure 8s—Push-Ups

Start with your feet shoulder-width apart and both hands on the ground. Circle around the cones, doing figure-8s and using your hands to guide you around the cones.

Quick Tips

Quick great endurance
  exercise
Shuffle the feet without
  crossing them

78. Knee-Ups

1. Stand with a split stance, holding your hands at shoulder level. Bring the back leg forward slowly and gently touch the spotter's hand to measure your mark. Return to the start position, ready to begin the movement.

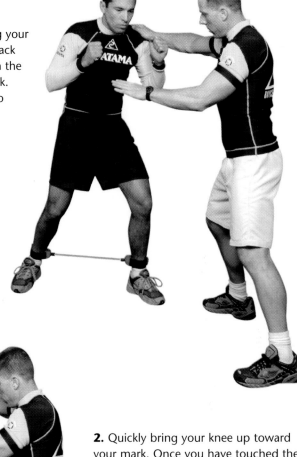

2. Quickly bring your knee up toward your mark. Once you have touched the mark, return to the starting position. Make sure to work both sides equally.

Quick Tips
Great way to develop hip-flexor
  strength
Can be done with or without a
  bungee cord

79. Lateral Hops

1. Position yourself sideways.

Quick Tips

Great for balance and explosive strength
Great for endurance and agility
Land on the balls of your feet
Bend at the knees when landing
Use a weight vest instead of the bungee if
  no spotter is available
Use different distances and thicknesses of
  bungee cord to vary the resistance
Concentrate on form and speed. If form
  suffers, stop the exercise and rest

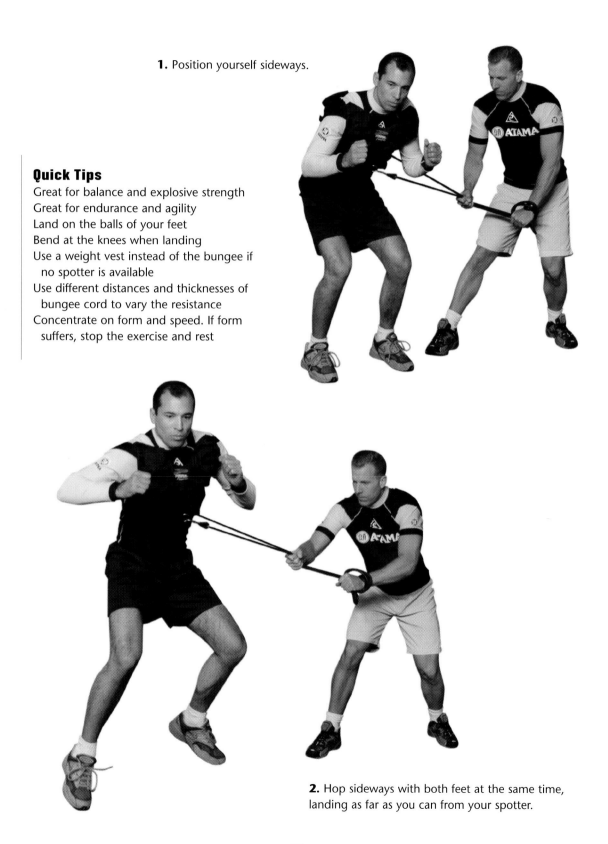

2. Hop sideways with both feet at the same time, landing as far as you can from your spotter.

80. Lateral Shuffle—Double Plate

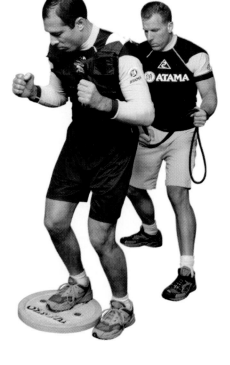

1. Place two sets of weight plates on the ground about two feet from each other. Your legs should be shoulder-width apart, with one foot on top of the plate.

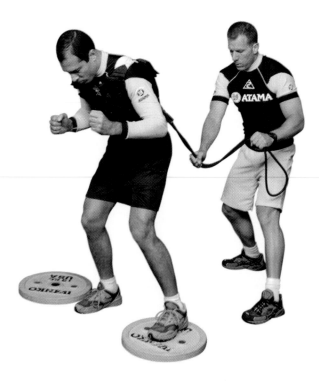

2. Pushing off that lead foot, jump to the middle of the plates with your trailing foot landing on top of the first weight plate.

Power Series PS

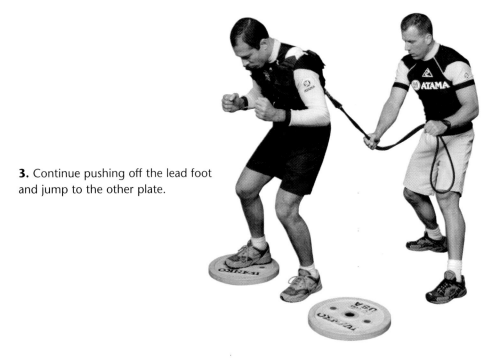

3. Continue pushing off the lead foot and jump to the other plate.

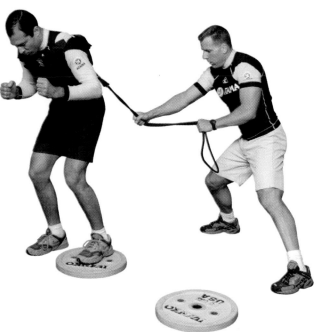

Quick Tips

Great for balance and explosive strength

Great for endurance and agility

Use a weight vest instead of the bungee if no spotter is available

Use different distances and thicknesses of bungee cord to vary the resistance

Concentrate on form and speed. If form suffers, stop the exercise and rest

4. Repeat until you get clear to the outside of the plates and return with the opposite motion. Adding more plates to make the stack higher will increase the difficulty of the exercise and add to your explosiveness.

81. Lateral Steps

1. Stand with legs at shoulder-width and one foot on top of the weight plates. The spotter pulls down on the harness.

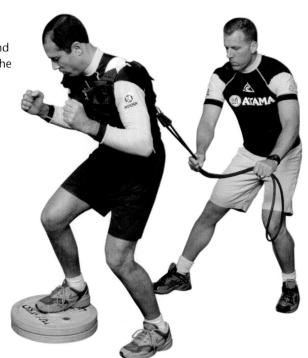

Quick Tips

Great for balance and explosive strength

Great for endurance and agility

Use a weight vest instead of the bungee if no spotter is available

Use different distances and thicknesses of bungee cord to vary the resistance

Concentrate on form and speed. If form suffers, stop the exercise and rest

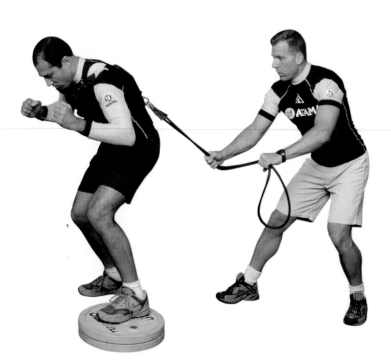

2. Pushing off the foot on the weights, jump over to the opposite landing, with your opposite foot on the plate, and repeat the motion. Adding more plates to make the stack higher will increase the difficulty of the exercise and add to your explosiveness.

82. Lateral Strides

1. Position yourself sideways from your spotter with feet shoulder-width apart.

Quick Tips

Great for balance and explosive
  strength
Great for endurance and agility
Use a weight vest instead of the bungee
  if no spotter is available
Use different distances and thicknesses
  of bungee cord to vary the resistance
Concentrate on form and speed. If form
  suffers, stop the exercise and rest

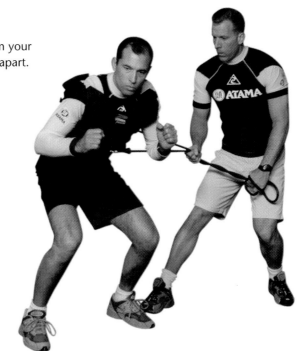

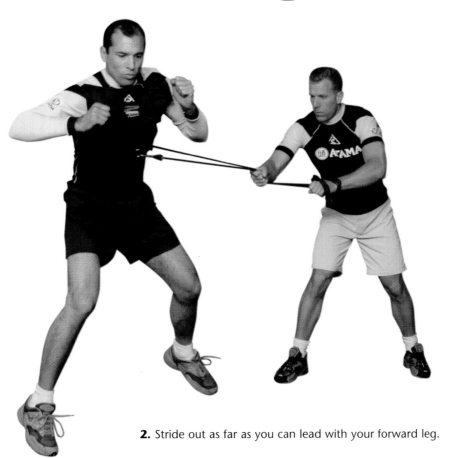

2. Stride out as far as you can lead with your forward leg.

83. Medicine Ball Toss—Chest

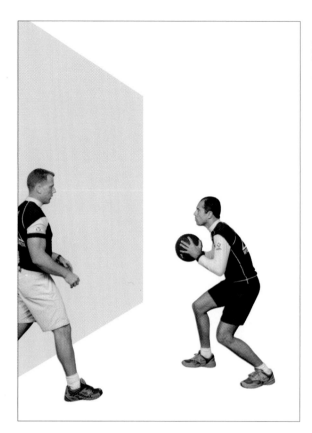

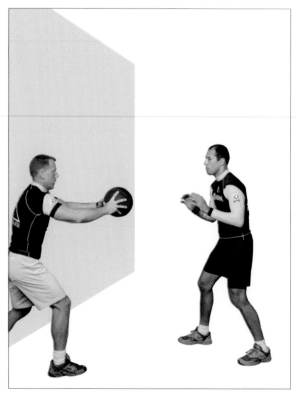

1. Stand in a split or parallel stance, slightly bending your legs in a ready position. Your arms should be flexed. Hold the medicine ball firmly with both hands at chest level.

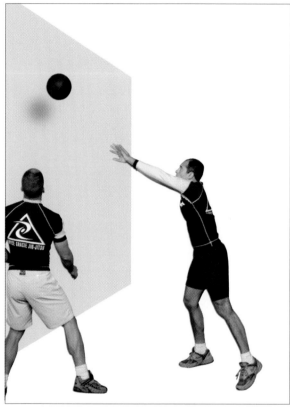

2. In a quick motion, extend your arms and legs to a split stance, throwing the medicine ball against the wall in an up plane.

Quick Tips
Can throw against a concrete wall for
  fast repetition benefiting conditioning
Good upper-body plyometric exercise
Intermediate/Advanced
Can use the split or parallel stance

3. Once you release the ball, quickly reposition your hands and feet and be ready to receive the medicine ball from the spotter and repeat the process.

84. Medicine Ball Toss—Overhead

1. Squat with your feet slightly wider than shoulder-width and your thighs parallel to the floor. Your arms are completely extended, holding the medicine ball down below the knees.

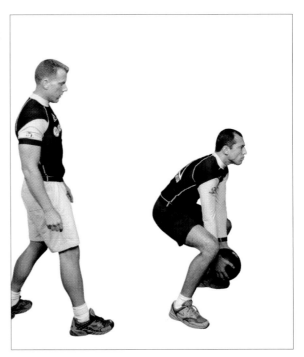

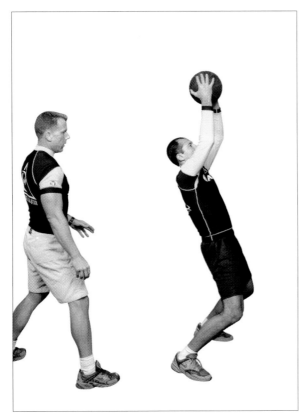

2. In a quick motion, extend your legs, bringing your arms up with great force. Your arms should be flexed up to slightly before the release point.

Quick Tips

Can throw against a concrete wall for
   fast repetition benefiting conditioning
Good upper-body plyometric exercise
Intermediate/Advanced
Great for upper-body explosiveness

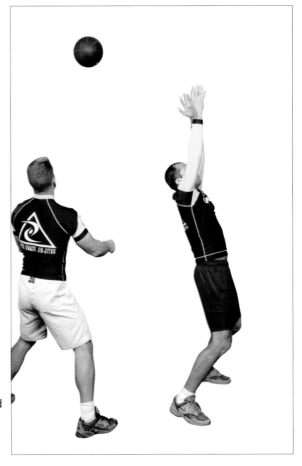

3. Upon releasing the medicine ball, your arms should be straight above your head. You should be up on your toes with a slight backward lean. Your spotter retrieves the medicine ball.

85. Power Lunges

1. Stand in a split stance with your hands at shoulder level. Your shoulders are positioned over your knees.

Quick Tips

Great for balance and explosive strength
Great for endurance and agility
Use a weight vest instead of the bungee
  if no spotter is available
Use different distances and thicknesses of
  bungee cord to vary the resistance
Concentrate on form and speed. If form
  suffers, stop the exercise and rest

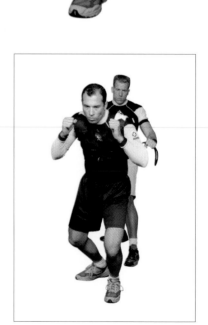

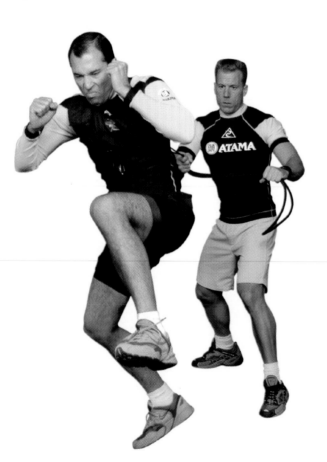

2. Quickly lunge forward, bringing your lead leg outward. For proper balance and strength, your knee should not go above your waist.

3. Land in balance and then reposition yourself for the next movement.

86. Power-Stride Jumps

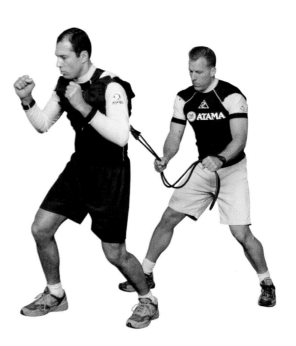

1. Start with a split stance.

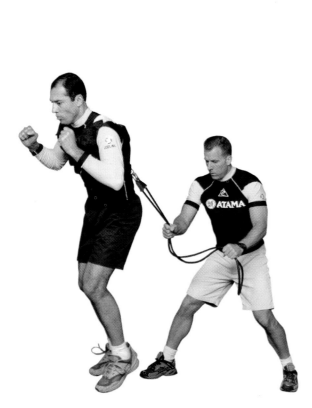

2. Push off your legs and jump up as you switch your feet.

Quick Tips

Great for balance and explosive strength

Great for endurance and agility

Use a weight vest instead of the bungee if no spotter is available

Use different distances and thicknesses of bungee cord to vary the resistance

Concentrate on form and speed. If form suffers, stop the exercise and rest.

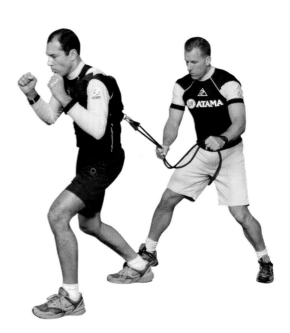

3. Land with the opposite foot at lead and repeat the motion.

87. Shoots

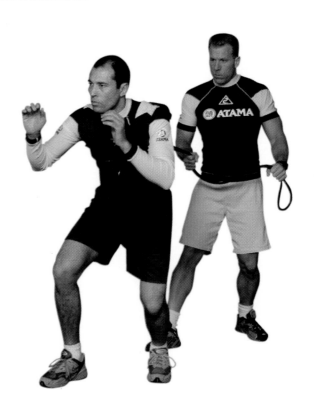

1. Stand in a split stance with your hands at shoulder level. Your shoulders are positioned over your knees.

Quick Tips
Great for balance and explosive strength
Great for endurance and agility
Use a weight vest instead of the bungee
 if no spotter is available
Use different distances and thicknesses
 of bungee cord to vary the resistance
Concentrate on form and speed. If form
 suffers, stop the exercise and rest

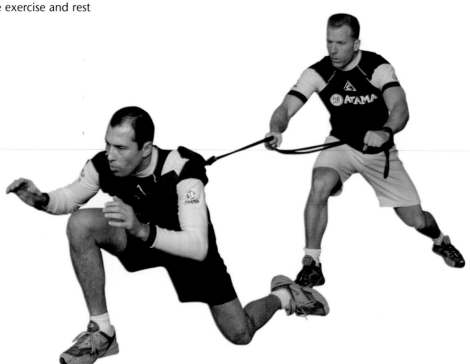

2. Take a deep stride with your lead leg as if you are shooting down into your opponent's legs.

88. Shuffle—Single Plate

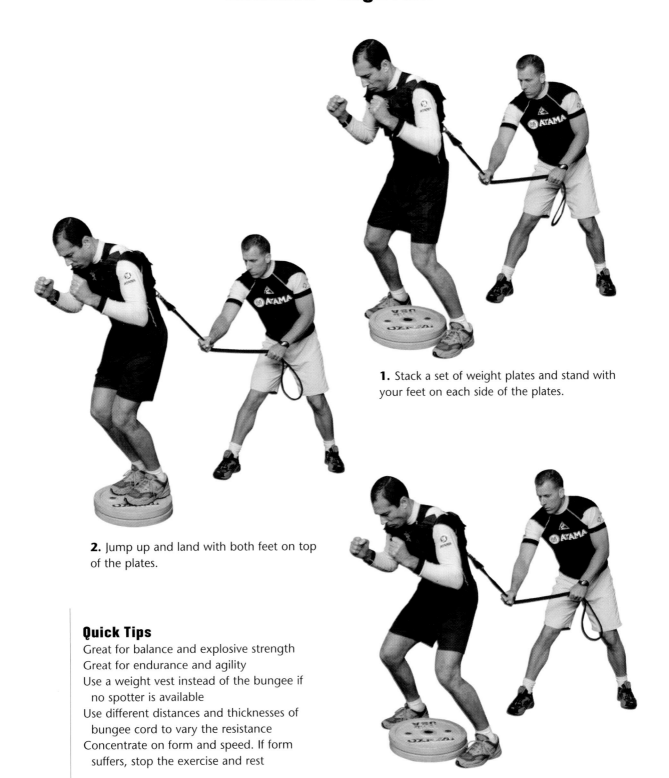

1. Stack a set of weight plates and stand with your feet on each side of the plates.

2. Jump up and land with both feet on top of the plates.

Quick Tips

Great for balance and explosive strength

Great for endurance and agility

Use a weight vest instead of the bungee if no spotter is available

Use different distances and thicknesses of bungee cord to vary the resistance

Concentrate on form and speed. If form suffers, stop the exercise and rest

3. Jump up and land with your feet on the sides of the plate stack.

89. Ski Jumps

1. Position yourself to one side of the bag with both feet firmly on the ground and parallel to the bag. Hands are held high at shoulder level.

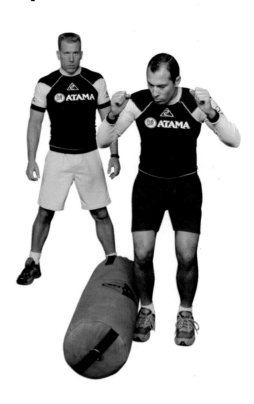

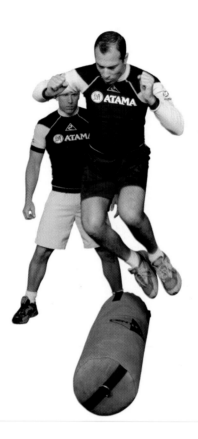

2. Slightly lean toward the opposite side of the bag and jump, pushing off the ground with both feet. Do quick lateral jumps.

Quick Tips

Land on the balls of your feet
Bend at the knees when landing
Intermediate/Advanced
Hold hands high
Good plyometric and endurance
  exercise

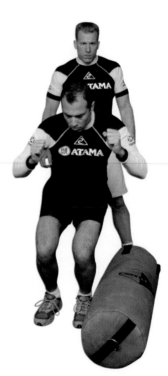

3. Land as close to the bag as possible and repeat the motion to the other side. Keep your hands high.

90. Static Wall Sit

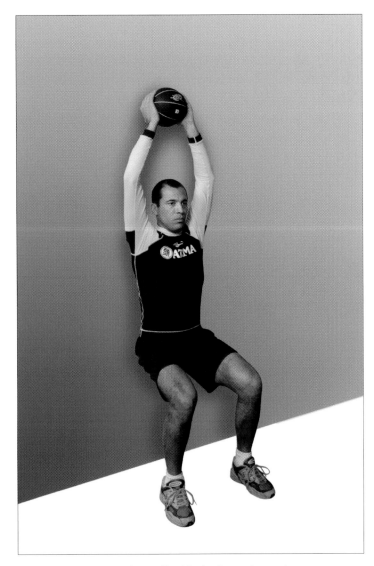

1. Stand up against the wall with the knees bent close to a 45-degree angle.

Quick Tips

Advanced: Hold a medicine ball above your head
   with arms stretched
Great way to develop mental strength as well

91. Squats—Medicine Ball or Plate

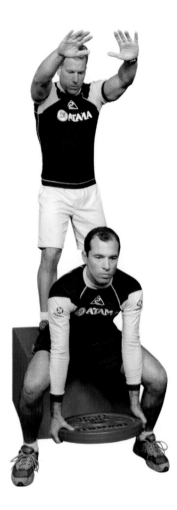

1. The spotter stands directly behind the lifter, with his hands held above the lifter. The lifter should take a shoulder-width stance with thighs parallel to the floor and keep the feet flat on the floor. Hold the medicine ball or plate firmly with both hands. The spotter can stand on a bench or box.

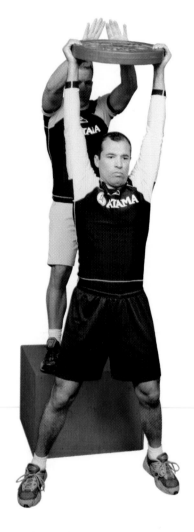

2. Before you begin the exercise, make sure the weight touches the spotter's hands at the highest point. With one quick but controlled motion, stand upright, raising the weight above your head. Once the weight has touched the spotter's hands, return to the starting position.

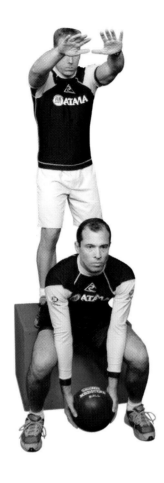

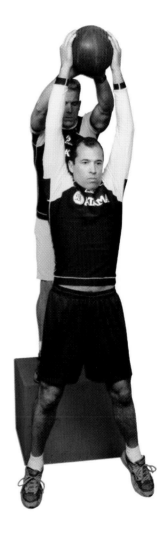

Quick Tips
Great endurance exercise
Intermediate/Advanced
Always use a spotter
Great total body exercise

92. Step-Ups—Barbell

1. Stand erect with one foot on the box. The grip is slightly wider than shoulder width. Angle the down leg slightly behind your body to enhance the up momentum.

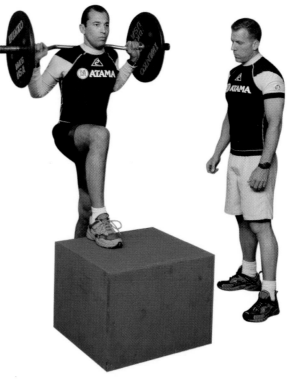

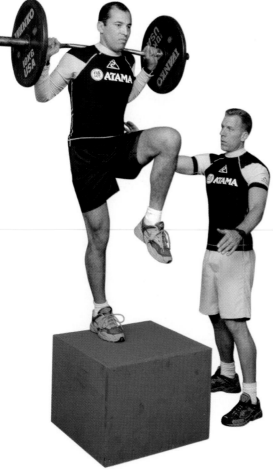

2. With one quick motion, bring the down leg up, using the up leg for power and balance. The spotter should provide a target for the knee by holding his hand out. Slowly step backward to the starting position.

Quick Tips
Make sure the box is steady
Intermediate/Advanced
Can use a flat bench instead of a box
Advanced: Barbell develops upper body balance as well

93. Step-Ups—Dumbbell

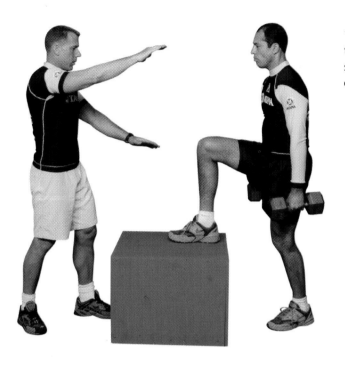

1. Stand erect with one foot on the box. Angle the down leg slightly behind your body to enhance the up momentum.

2. With one quick motion, bring the down leg up, using the up leg for power and balance. The spotter should provide a target for the knee by holding his hand out. Slowly step backward to the starting position.

Quick Tips
Make sure the box is steady
Intermediate/Advanced
Can use a flat bench instead of a box

— PART THREE —

Putting It All Together

Most exercise routines have a goal of increasing power or endurance, but not both. To build power, you reduce the repetitions and increase the weights. To improve endurance, you increase the reps. What makes the *Superfit* system unique is that we combine strength, endurance, and power training to make a complete athlete by using different phases of training. That is, for two weeks you may be in a power phase, and then for two weeks you could be in the endurance phase, and then two weeks prior to competition you combine the two to get optimum performance at that event.

Whether or not you are an elite athlete like Royce, what we try to do in our system is give you the tools you need to perform in your real world, whatever that world may be. For Royce, that may mean being able to fight for ninety minutes against an elite opponent in Pride, while for someone else it may be to lift boxes at the warehouse, to climb rock walls, or just to be healthy, physically fit, and able to meet life's challenges with confidence. The program will enable you to become functionally strong in the core.

Don't underestimate the importance of organization in your routine. Even if you are a beginner, you need to be organized and have a program so you improve each day. Don't just go out there and do what you feel like doing on a given day. Get a game plan and enough specific guidance so that you know what you need to do to achieve your specific goal. This system gives you a roadmap; after you start to understand it, you will be able to adapt it to your own changing needs.

One of the major differences between the *Superfit* system and other types of workouts is that *Superfit* doesn't divide the training week into specific days for legs or back or chest. We aren't trying to show you how to become a bodybuilder or to sculpt your body to some standard. Rather, our goal is to make you a better athlete, and athletes and fighters use all their body parts in training and when they fight. So our workouts tax your entire body every session. They are much more demanding! Sure, some days you might do more leg work than others, but overall the workouts are balanced because the tool you use is a single body, not a bunch of parts. In the *Superfit* system, all six types of exercises described earlier have been carefully integrated to help you develop the functional power you need.

Additionally, when your workouts concentrate on one specific body part at a time, you do not put your cardio system through its maximum range. What you need to do is to use all your body parts each day to get your system used to supporting your whole body, which will further develop your conditioning. Endurance is a key consideration in the martial arts. Many fights are decided by who tires first.

You need to develop the strength and endurance to maintain a weight program, but you also must develop coordination. You may start to realize that your body was not balanced, that, for instance, your left side was weaker than your right side—a realization that comes when you are doing dumbbell bench presses and one side does not respond as well as the other. This learning curve continues as long as you are doing an exercise program. Some martial artists like to start their program by gaining bulk, doing a lot of weightlifting to gain strength, and then add explosiveness by doing the plyometrics. Then they drop the weight routine down a little and add endurance. This sequence is called tapering. You start with the heavier, slower exercises, then as you get near the event, you start to taper the weight training and increase the explosion/endurance workouts. That way, you develop your endurance while still maintaining the functional power you have gained.

A common mistake athletes make, especially at the intermediate level, is to train hard all the way to the day before competition, leaving them nothing to deliver when it counts. They left it all in the gym. That mistake also leads to injuries, because when you push your body too hard and without a proper taper, you overstress your muscular system and it starts to break down. This happens even at the highest levels of competition. You see it a lot in boxing, where a fighter overtrains, gets to the fight flat, and gets hurt in the ring. Proper tapering is a science; while we offer general guidelines, it is up to each individual to understand what works best for him.

Most of your gains will come in the early stage of fitness training, because everything is brand new to your body. Since you are seeing such big results so quickly, it will be tempting to overdo it. You think, "Well, if I got this result with 50 reps, if I do 100 reps I'll get twice the result!" But that is not the case. It is vital that you restrain yourself, introducing your body gradually to the exercises to familiarize your joints, muscles, and tendons with the movements and resistance. Typically, most injuries and gains occur in the early phases of training. Therefore, it is very important to take it slow so you avoid injuries that can set you back tremendously.

Focus

The challenge is to have a program and a series of exercises that are not dull or boring. You must not only get the benefits of the work but actually enjoy doing them. This helps you stay focused. If you do exercises that do not challenge you, like machine exercises, then your workout will become all work and no play, but when you do things like the plyometric exercises, you are constantly challenging yourself to do them properly. You can't just go through the motions; you have to pay attention to what you're doing and get engaged in the process. These types of exercises not only make the workout seem faster and more entertaining, but they also simulate fighting much more closely.

One of the difficulties for people in fitness training is to remain focused on the program and not lose interest, because as you advance in your workouts, the gains get smaller and smaller. The payoff is less obvious, so people sometimes lose interest or think that the program is not working because they got used to constant, observable improvements and changes in their body. One way to combat workout fatigue is to change your workouts regularly. The human body is a very efficient machine and it adapts quickly to everything. When you do one program with the same exercises for a long time, your body adjusts, and as a consequence, you get less benefit from the same exercises. So you need to change things up. Our workouts are designed to give you maximum flexibility in determining your own course of training. Once you have mastered the basic workout, you are encouraged to experiment by replacing the exercises presented in the workouts with others from the same family. For example, you might remove the box jumps (a plyometric exercise) from your routine and replace them with lateral jumps (also a plyo exercise). Use the icons that mark each exercise category to help you swap similar exercises.

Another thing you can change is the order of the exercises. Even a simple modification like that can send your "machine" into a readjustment period and increase the challenge once again. Although typically you should begin a workout with the harder exercises, by simply changing the order of the exercises you are going to create a new challenge—not only for your body but for your mind as well. The next step beyond that is to change to a different program, like going "back" to the beginner series and adapting it to your new level (by increasing the weight load or repetitions). By doing that you are going to once again disturb your "machine" and challenge it to progress and improve. This actually reenergizes your whole system.

Another variation we are fond of is, instead of doing all the sets of the first exercise, then moving on to the second, and so on, take the first three exercises and do one set of each. Then do one set of each again. Continue doing this until you have completed the first three exercises, then move on to the next group of three and do the same thing. This varies your workout and challenges your muscles in a new way. It makes particular sense for martial artists, who in competition are called on to do many different moves in quick succession, rather than the same move again and again.

Fight Preparation

Royce likes three to four months to prepare for a fight. The first thing he does is to stop everything—traveling, seminars, everything—and just stay home and eat well and rest. He starts concentrating on his opponent, stepping up his training and physical preparation.

> **Royce:** I need all my energy to do my training. I do a technical training in the morning that lasts 60 to 90 minutes, then we do a hard training in the afternoon. But when I say hard training, I don't mean an all-out brawl. My training is best described as reckless control because I cannot afford to get injured. When a show depends on my presence and the organizers are counting on my presence as their top star, I can't go to them and say, "Oh well, I can't fight because I got injured training! You guys understand, right?" They won't! I fought in a Pride Dynamite event in 2002 in Japan that had

91,000 spectators—imagine if I hadn't shown up because I got a last minute injury! So part of my preparation and part of being a professional is to protect myself so that I can show up and fight when I agreed to fight!

Working together, we start with gaining strength and bulk. Although it is very hard to add bulk to Royce because he is naturally super lean, we still do it. We start with overall strength and don't worry about his conditioning, even though conditioning is always a part of the workout. As we get closer to the fight, we taper down and start adding more cardio with the strength. Ideally, you bulk up and try to create leaner mass as you get closer to a fight without losing the gained strength. Of course, that isn't easy and many times is impossible, but if we achieve a 15 percent gain in power and strength after the first phase, then as we get leaner and better conditioned in the second phase, he may lose some of his strength but still end up 12 percent stronger overall than when he first started. We also add explosiveness as we get closer to the fight. Each phase lasts four to six weeks. The first phase concentrates on strength gain, the second focuses on strength with conditioning, and the third phase is a lean explosion and agility phase, which is where the plyometrics workouts come in. We start working the clock a little more and our rests become more structured—usually 30 seconds.

At this point, we also use more interval training to increase Royce's ability to perform during a fight. Basically, interval training structures a workout using intervals of exercise and rest periods. The intervals may be set by time, in which case you might work out for one minute and rest for one minute, or by heartbeat, in which case you might work out for one minute and then rest until your heartbeat reaches a predetermined number. In Royce's own plyometric routine, he exercises for 15 seconds and rests for 45 seconds. He does three sets of six exercises, for a total of 18 minutes.

Royce: You need to customize your conditioning to meet your goals. I prepare myself for the long haul, so I like to do the workouts that keep my heart rate high for a long period of time—like the plyometric or power series—in an interval training setting with very short rest periods. Many people like to get their heart rates up, but only keep it up for a short period of time, like two minutes. Then they go, "ufff," and rest to let the heart rate go back down. I prefer to keep my rate high for long periods, depending on the length of the rounds I expect to fight. Of course, I like to fight with no time limits, but nowadays that doesn't happen very often. It's more realistic to expect that I'll have 10- to 15-minute rounds, so I train with a high heart rate for 20- to 30-minute intervals with short rests between. I never let the heart rate go completely down to full rest!

It's easy to be in good shape and have low body fat, but still tire quickly. I strive for the endurance of a marathon runner. I like to go for 90-minute bike rides around the Palos Verdes peninsula where there are lots of steep hills to climb, keeping my heart rate at 180 to 190. My secret is that my training demands this high rate for a long time, so my rate of recovery is also very high. As I am riding, if I hit a flat area, my heart rate drops down to 120 after one minute. Others train for a sprint, and then at the end of the round they are dead. I don't train for a short explosion; I train to be able to maintain the pace indefinitely.

If you aren't training for a particular event, you need to take breaks from your routine, so you don't burn out. As we mentioned in the introduction, after four to six weeks of training, you need to take an active rest for at least two weeks. Active rest can be any exercise that is unrelated to your normal workout routine but that still keeps your muscles working. Raquetball, tennis, basketball, and bike riding are all good examples of active rest.

Now here is a secret: When you start back up with your weight training routine after two weeks of active rest, start at a lower level than the one you finished with and build back up. Many people err and injure themselves by restarting their workout program at the same weight and intensity at which they stopped. That is a mistake. After the active rest phase, you need to build back up to your best level, which will happen fairly quickly, but don't just jump back into your maximum performance.

Mental Preparation

Although *Superfit* is about your physical training routine, we would be remiss if we didn't address the issue of mental training. No martial artists ever became champion by being physically perfect but mentally weak. To win matches, you need a sound body *and* mind.

Royce is as famous for his mental toughness as anyone on the planet, so let's let him tell us how he does it:

> **Royce:** Visualize the fight. Three days before the fight, I get my coaches, my dad, and my brothers. I get one of them in a room, dim the lights, start doing a relaxation breathing, and we begin to talk. I describe what I see in the fight. I visualize it. I will say, "The bell rings and I walk toward him," and my dad will ask a question: "Does he have his guard up? Are his hands up? Does he want to strike?" Depending on the answer I give, we go through the scenarios and options. I see the fight going this way, but if my opponent does this, then we will do that. If he does that, then we will do this, and so forth. Visualizing the fight always helps. I talk to the coaches so they know I am confident, and they know what I am thinking. We make sure we are synchronized and are all thinking as one.
>
> Another great thing I do is to imagine what my opponent can do to me. Many times people have asked me who my toughest opponent was, and my answer is: the one inside my head. The opponent inside my head is 6' 7" and 350 pounds, 4 percent body fat, flexible, with great endurance. He has two heads and four arms. I make him invincible and try to see how I would defeat him and what he could do to me! To beat the best you have to plan for the worst.

You can visualize fights during your everyday training and at completely different times. Some days you can't practice, but you can still perform these mental exercises to stay mentally sharp. You can also do them to correct a problem that you may have in certain positions or situations. Often, when you are working out or training you are too busy concentrating on the now to think of correcting or even noticing what you are doing wrong. However, if you have a certain level of ability and understanding, you may be able to see for yourself what your mistake is by visualizing the situation at some other time. Sometimes you can't do it alone; then you need your instructor's help.

Royce: By the time I get to a fight I am very calm, because I know that I am prepared to fight forever. At Pride Grand-Prix, I fought six 15-minute rounds against Sakuraba! If you are prepared to fight forever, you have good technique, you understand the game, and you have already prepared for most of the variables and for your opponent, then you can relax prior to the fight, because you know you are ready. The problem for some people is that they don't have enough experience to understand the game, or they are not in their best shape when they get to the fight, or they don't believe in their technical skills and worry about their opponent's skills. These uncertainties add a lot of pressure and make them get tired even faster. Imagine that you show up to a fight and the rounds are 15 minutes long, but during the training you were getting tired at the end of 10 minutes. You will now be under a huge amount of pressure to finish the fight fast because you already know that you don't have enough stamina to get through many rounds. So you will spend even more of your energy to press the action for a fast decision, worrying the whole time. You know that with each passing minute you are getting closer to the "empty tank," and that knowledge will take you out of your game, which will tire you even faster and force you to take risks you normally wouldn't, and so on.

If you know all this coming into a fight—that you know you didn't prepare well for one reason or another—then several hours before you go in the ring you will already be using up energy; your heart rate will be high. With me, one hour before the fight my heart beat is only 65 beats per minute; just before walking in the ring my heart rate goes 78–80. I am as normal as ever, concentrating on my performance!

The other piece of mental training is discipline. To develop discipline is almost impossible; you either have it or you don't. The same thing with determination. These are the attributes that separate the winners from the talkers. You must have discipline and determination to reach the top. If you don't have them, you can get a coach to help you develop them. You need to associate yourself with someone you respect, who will be your conscience and get you to do the things you won't do on your own, but that still may not be enough. To reach the top levels, you need to have a burning fire inside of you, and no coach can provide that. Some great coaches will find that fire inside you, where you couldn't locate it yourself, but it must be present somewhere within you if you expect to become a champion.

The Workouts

As we've said, don't do too much too soon! Start slow, and work your way up into championship form. We recommend that beginners start working out three nonconsecutive days a week, for example, Monday, Wednesday, and Friday. As you get to the intermediate level, you should be at four days a week, say Monday, Tuesday, Thursday, and Friday. The advanced practitioner should move up to five or six days a week. Nobody should do seven days a week!

The beginner and intermediate workouts are four weeks long and should be followed by a two-week active rest break. The advanced workout is designed to be six weeks long—the two weeks described in the routine below plus four weeks of a stepped-up intermediate routine—and should also be followed by two weeks of active rest. After the rest interval, proceed to the next fitness level if you feel you have achieved it. During each four- or six-week interval, increase the load (weights) as you see necessary, always keeping in mind the rule of thumb of having enough weight so that you can barely do the last rep.

As mentioned earlier, once you are ready to progress from beginner to intermediate or intermediate to advanced, keep in mind that a weight adjustment may be necessary, and even desired, to acclimate yourself to the new routine. So on your first day at the intermediate level, for instance, if the routine feels like it is too much, try stepping back on the weights. Perhaps at the end of the beginner's level you were doing lateral raises with 30 pounds on each arm, but the intermediate routine requires a few more reps from you, and the extra requirements are getting to be too much. It may be the time to lower the load for the exercises, even if only temporarily, so that your body can get adjusted to the new demands.

If you are an advanced practitioner or a beginner or intermediate who wants to stay at your present workout level for another four weeks before advancing, remember to modify your routine. The workouts at all levels are designed with this flexibility in mind. As noted previously, if you need to alter your workout to fight workout fatigue, you can modify your routine in three distinct ways. First, you can always alter the sequence of the specified exercises. Second, you can increase the difficulty of a given exercise. For example, the free weights exercise "front raises" can be executed with the barbell, dumbbells, plates, or isolaterally. If you are a beginner, start with the easiest options (dumbbells, then isolaterally with dumbbells). As you get more advanced, proceed to the more difficult options (plates and barbell). Finally, you can use the icons to substitute one exercise for another in the same family. In the intermediate workout, for instance, week 1 day 3 calls for plyometrics. You could easily replace one or several of the plyometric exercises with others from the plyometrics category in part 2 to design a new workout! The Medicine Ball Walk (74.1) could be replaced with Medicine Ball Ground Work—One Hand (71). You could even turbocharge into a Power Series exercise, such as Cones Workout (77). The icons will also help advanced practitioners, who are directed after the first two weeks to go back and use the intermediate four-week program, adding an exercise of the same group to each day's routine.

To get the maximum benefits of the *Superfit* program, you should end each workout with the cardiovascular conditioning exercises that are specified. However, there are times when this will not be possible, and in those cases it is okay to do the cardio part at a different time. In either case, don't forget to warm up and stretch!

Each line in the workouts below represents a complete exercise. For example, in the line

FW **Pullovers—Dumbbell (36):** 10; 10; 10

the first item is the title (Pullovers—Dumbbell), and the number in parenthesis (36 in this case) refers to the exercise number in part 2. If a title is not followed by a number, we assume you need no explanation of the exercise. Such is the case, for example, with push-ups. The numbers that follow the colon are the repetitions for each set. The line above specifies 3 sets of 10 repetitions, meaning that you would do 10 reps of the exercise for the first set, rest for a pre-established period, then do 2 more sets of 10 reps each followed by proper rest to complete that exercise before proceeding to the next exercise of that day's workout. The icon on each line will help you exchange exercises when you are ready to modify your workout.

Proper rest intervals depend on each individual. For beginners, we recommend between one and two minutes rest between sets and at least two minutes between exercises. If after two minutes you don't feel ready to go on, you should wait and collect yourself before proceeding. Conversely, if after 30 seconds you feel ready to rock, then go ahead. It is important that you learn to adjust the rest time to best fit your body and fitness level. Another way to set rest intervals, of course, is to use a heart beat monitor and set a desired heart beat level of rest. In other words, you set say 100 hbpm (heart beats per minute) as your rest level, then you would do the exercise and upon finishing it, rest until your heart beat gets down to that level. This is a more advanced way but it is a very effective method of pushing your limits, especially in plyometric exercises and interval training.

BEGINNER WORKOUT BW

3 days/week

At the end of the four weeks, take two weeks of active rest doing an activity that you prefer—like bicycling, running, swimming, or playing tennis—before you advance to the intermediate workout. If you feel you are not ready to proceed to the intermediate workout routine yet, then repeat the four weeks in the beginner workout and replace at least one exercise in each workout day with another one of the same family or simply alter the exercise order to challenge your system a little more.

Week 1
Day 1

Warm-Up

CC Jump Rope (7): 45 seconds; 45 seconds; 45 seconds
    or
FW Lunges (body weight only) (31): 10 reps per side; 10 reps per side; 10 reps per side

Stretch

GSR Gracie Stretch Routine

Strength Training—Chest and Back

FW Upright Row—Dumbbell (53): 10; 10; 10
    or
FW Pullovers—Dumbbell (36): 10; 10; 10

PL Push-Ups: 10–15; 10–15; 10–15

FW Bench Press—Barbell (14): 10; 10; 10

Strength Training—Legs

FW Squats (body weight only) (45): 15–20; 15–20; 15–20

Abdominals

AB Bench Crunches (1): 15–20; 15–20; 15–20

Cardiovascular Conditioning

CC Steady Run or Jog (12): 10–12 minutes

CC Lateral Cone Touches (8): 20 seconds, rest 1:30; 20 seconds, rest 1:30 ; 20 seconds, rest 1:30

Week 1
Day 2

Warm-Up

CC Jump Rope (7): 45 seconds; 45 seconds; 45 seconds
or
PL Step-Ups—Body Weight (76): 8–10 per leg; 8–10 per leg; 8–10 per leg

Stretch

GSR Gracie Stretch Routine

Strength Training—Shoulders

FW Lateral Raise—Dumbbell (28): 10; 10; 10
or
FW Front Raise—Barbell (17): 10; 10; 10

FW Shoulder Shrugs—Dumbbell (43): 10; 10; 10

FW Military Press—Barbell (32): 10; 10; 10

Strength Training—Plyometrics

PL Box Jumps (use small box) (66): 8; 8; 8

PS Power-Stride Jumps (86): 10–16; 10–16; 10–16

Cardiovascular Conditioning

CC Steady Run or Jog (12): 10–12 minutes

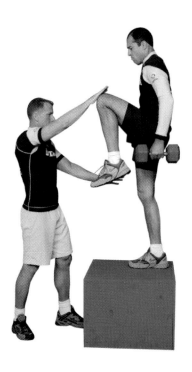

Week 1

Day 3

Warm-Up

CC Jump Rope (7): 45 seconds; 45 seconds; 45 seconds
   or
FW Lunges (body weight only) (31): 10 reps per side; 10 reps per side; 10 reps per side

Stretch

GSR Gracie Stretch Routine

Strength Training—Chest/Back/Legs

FW Pullovers—Dumbbell (36): 10; 10; 10

PL Push-Ups: 10–15; 10–15; 10–15

FW Bench Press—Barbell (14): 10; 10; 10

FW High Pull—Dumbbell (22): 10; 10; 10

PS Squats—Medicine Ball or Plate (91): 15–20; 15–20; 15–20

Abdominals

AB Bench Crunches (1): 15–20; 15–20; 15–20

Cardiovascular Conditioning

CC Steady Run or Jog (12): 12 minutes

CC Lateral Cone Touches (8): 20 seconds; 20 seconds; 20 seconds

Week 2
Day 1

Warm-Up

(CC) Steady Run or Jog (12): 5 minutes

Stretch

(GSR) Gracie Stretch Routine

Strength Training—Plyometrics

(PS) Cones Workout (Figure 8s—Push-Ups)(77.2): 15 seconds; 15 seconds; 15 seconds

(PL) Medicine Ball Ground Work—One Hand (71): 15 seconds; 15 seconds; 15 seconds

(PS) Medicine Ball Toss—Chest (83): 8–12; 8–12; 8–12

(FW) Rice Grabs (56): 30 seconds; 30 seconds; 30 seconds

Abdominals

(AB) Roll-Ups—Abdominal (3): 15–20; 15–20; 15–20

Cardiovascular Conditioning

(CC) Sprints (13): 8–10 sprints, 100 yards each. Walk back to starting point.

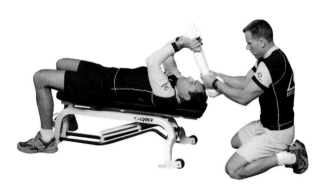

Week 2

Day 2

Warm-Up

FW Rice Grabs (56): 30 seconds; 30 seconds; 30 seconds

PS Ski Jumps (89): 12–15; 12–15; 12–15

Stretch

GSR Gracie Stretch Routine

Strength Training—Shoulders and Legs

FW Lateral Raise—Dumbbell (28): 10; 10; 10

FW Front Raise—Barbell (17): 10; 10; 10

FW Shoulder Shrugs—Dumbbell (43): 10; 10; 10

FW Military Press—Barbell (32): 10; 10; 10; 10

FW Upright Row—Barbell (52): 10; 10; 10

FW Squats—Dumbbell (45): 10; 10; 10; 10

Abdominals

AB Roll-Ups—Abdominals (3): 15–20; 15–20; 15–20

Cardiovascular Conditioning

CC

Steady Run or Jog (12): 15–18 minutes

Week 2
Day 3

Warm-Up

FW Rice Grabs (56): 30 seconds; 30 seconds; 30 seconds

FW Lunges (body weight only) (31): 10 reps per side; 10 reps per side; 10 reps per side

Stretch

GSR Gracie Stretch Routine

Strength Training—Chest and Back

FW Pullovers—Towel (37): 12; 12; 12

FW Bench Press—Dumbbell (15): 10; 10; 10; 10

FW High Pull—Dumbbell (22): 8; 8; 8

FW Incline Press—Dumbbell (25): 10; 10; 10

FW Pull-Ups: 4–8; 4–8; 4–8

Abdominals

AB Bench Crunches (1): 15–20; 15–20; 15–20

AB Roll-Ups—Abdominal (3): 15–20; 15–20; 15–20

Cardiovascular Conditioning

CC Steady Run or Jog (12): 15–18 minutes

CC Lateral Cone Touches (8): 20 seconds; 20 seconds; 20 seconds

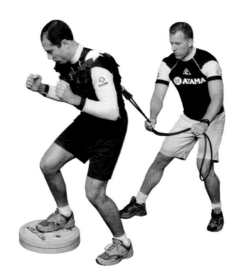

Week 3
Day 1

Warm-Up

FW Roll-Ups—Wrist (40): 10; 10; 10

PS Power-Stride Jumps (86): 10–16; 10–16; 10–16

Stretch

GSR Gracie Stretch Routine

Strength Training—Shoulders and Legs

FW Front Raise—Barbell (17): 10; 10; 10

FW Lateral Raise—Dumbbell (28): 10; 10; 10

FW Military Press—Dumbbell (33): 10; 10; 8; 8

FW Upright Row—Plate (54): 10; 10; 10

FW Lunges (body weight only) (31): 10 reps per side; 10; reps per side; 10 reps per side

FW Straight-Leg Dead Lifts—Dumbbell (49): 10; 10; 10

Cardiovascular Conditioning

CC Sprints (13): 8–10 sprints, 100 yards each. Walk back to starting point.

Week 3
Day 2

Warm-Up

CC Steady Run or Jog (12): 5 minutes

Stretch

GSR Gracie Stretch Routine

Strength Training—Plyometrics

PS Cones Workout (Figure 8s—Push-Ups) (77.2): 15 seconds; 15 seconds; 15 seconds

PL Medicine Ball Toss—Flat Bench (73): 10–15; 10–15; 10–15

PL Lateral Jumps—Short Way (70): 12–16; 12–16; 12–16

CC Jump Rope (7): 45 seconds; 45 seconds; 45 seconds

PL Medicine Ball Ground Work—Two Hands (72): 20 seconds; 20 seconds; 20 seconds

Abdominals

AB Roll-Ups—Abdominal (3): 12–15; 12–15; 12–15

Cardiovascular Conditioning

CC Steady Run or Jog (12): 15–18 minutes

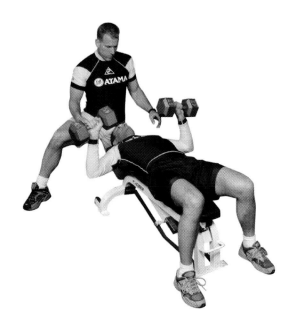

Week 3

Day 3

Warm-Up

CC Jump Rope (7): 45 seconds; 45 seconds; 45 seconds
    or
FW Lunges (body weight only) (31): 10 reps per side; 10 reps per side; 10 reps per side

Stretch

GSR Gracie Stretch Routine

Strength Training—Chest/Back/Legs

FW Row—Dumbbell (41): 10; 10; 10
    or
FW Pullovers—Towel (37): 12; 12; 12

PL Push-Ups: 10–15; 10–15; 10–15

FW Bench Press—Barbell (14): 10; 10; 10

PS Squats—Medicine Ball or Plate (91): 15–20; 15–20; 15–20

Abdominals

AB Bench Crunches (1): 15–20; 15–20; 15–20

Cardiovascular Conditioning

CC Steady Run or Jog (12): 15–20 minutes

Week 4
Day 1

Warm-Up

FW **Rice Grabs (56):** 30 seconds; 30 seconds; 30 seconds

FW **Lunges (body weight only) (31):** 10 reps per side; 10 reps per side; 10 reps per side

Stretch

GSR Gracie Stretch Routine

Strength Training—Chest and Back

FW **Pullovers—Dumbbell (36):** 10; 10; 10

FW **Incline Press—Dumbbell (25):** 10; 10; 10

FW **High Pull—Dumbbell (22):** 8; 8; 8

FW **Bench Press—Dumbbell (15):** 10; 10; 10; 10

FW **Pull-Ups:** 4–8; 4–8; 4–8

Abdominals

AB **Bench Crunches (1):** 15–20; 15–20; 15–20

AB **Roll-Ups—Abdominal (3):** 15–20; 15–20; 15–20

Cardiovascular Conditioning

CC **Steady Run or Jog (12):** 15–18 minutes

CC **Lateral Cone Touches (8):** 20 seconds; 20 seconds; 20 seconds

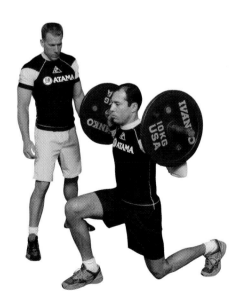

Week 4

Day 2

Warm-Up

CC Run in Place (9) or Steady Run or Jog (12): 5 minutes

Stretch

GSR Gracie Stretch Routine

Strength Training—Grip and Shoulders

PL Medicine Ball Ground Work—Two Hands (72): 12–15 reps; 12–15 reps; 12–15 reps

FW Rice Grabs (56): 30 seconds; 30 seconds; 30 seconds

PS Medicine Ball Toss—Chest (83): 8–12; 8–12; 8–12

FW Lateral Raise—Dumbbell Seated (29): 10; 10; 10

FW Upright Row—Plate (54): 10; 10; 10

FW Shoulder Shrugs—Dumbbell (Hands-on) (43a): 10; 10; 10

FW Military Press—Dumbbell (33): 10; 10; 8; 8

Abdominals

FW Good Mornings* (46): 12; 12; 12

Cardiovascular Conditioning

CC Sprints (13): 8–10 sprints, 100 yards each. Walk back to starting point.

*While considered free weight exercises, Good Mornings provide an excellent abdominal workout too.

Week 4
Day 3

Warm-Up

FW Roll-Ups—Wrist (40): 8; 8; 8

PS Power-Stride Jumps (86): 12–15; 12–15; 12–15

Stretch

GSR Gracie Stretch Routine

Strength Training—Chest/Back/Legs

PL Push-Ups: 12–15; 12–15; 12–15

FW Row—Dumbbell (41): 10; 10; 10

FW Bench Press—Narrow Grip Barbell (16): 10; 10; 10

FW Pullovers—Towel (37): 12; 12; 12

FW Squats—Dumbbell (45): 10; 10; 10; 10

PL Step-Ups—Body Weight (76): 10–12 per leg; 10–12 per leg; 10–12 per leg

Cardiovascular Conditioning

CC Steady Run or Jog (12): 15–18 minutes

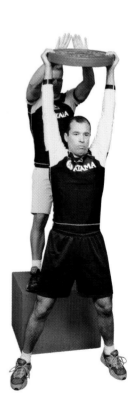

INTERMEDIATE WORKOUT IW

4 days/week

At the end of the four-week routine described here, take two weeks of active rest doing an activity that you enjoy—like bicycling, running, swimming, or playing tennis—before you move on to the advanced workout. If you feel you are not ready to proceed to the advanced workout routine yet, then repeat the four weeks in the intermediate workout and replace at least one exercise in each workout day with another one of the same family or simply alter the exercise order to challenge your system a little more.

Week 1

Day 1

Warm-Up

FW Reverse Hypers (47): 10; 10; 10

FW Good Mornings (46): 10; 10; 10

CC Jump Rope (7): 60 seconds; 60 seconds; 60 seconds

Stretch

GSR Gracie Stretch Routine

Strength Training—Chest/Back/Legs

FW Straight-Leg Dead Lifts—Dumbbell (49): 10; 10; 10

FW Squats—Dumbbell (45): 10; 10; 10; 10

PL Box Jumps—One Leg (67): 8–10; 8–10; 8–10

ISO Bench Press—Isolateral (57): 10; 8; 8; 6; 6

FW Pullovers—Dumbbell (36): 8; 8; 8; 8

ISO Incline Press—Isolateral (59): 8; 8; 8; 8

FW Towel Pull-Ups (51): 6–8; 6–8; 6–8

Abdominals

AB Bench Crunches (1): 20; 20; 20

Cardiovascular Conditioning

CC Steady Run or Jog (12): 5–8 minutes

CC Sprints (13): 4–6 sprints, 200 yards each. Walk back to starting point.

Week 1
Day 2

Warm-Up

FW Rice Grabs (56): 45 seconds; 45 seconds; 45 seconds

PL Step-Ups—Body Weight (quick feet) (76): 25 seconds; 25 seconds; 25 seconds; 25 seconds

Stretch

GSR Gracie Stretch Routine

Strength Training—Shoulders

ISO Front Raise—Isolateral (58): 10; 10; 10; 10

ISO Lateral Raise—Isolateral (60): 10; 10; 10; 10

ISO Military Press—Isolateral (61): 8; 8; 6; 6

FW High Pull—Dumbbell (22): 6; 6; 6; 6

FW Shoulder Shrugs—Dumbbell (Hands-on) (43a): 10; 10; 10; 10

FW Upright Row—Barbell (52): 8; 8; 8; 8

Abdominals

AB V-Ups (6): 12–15; 12–15; 12–15; 12–15

Cardiovascular Conditioning

CC Steady Run or Jog (12): 5–8 minutes

CC Sprints (13): 4–6 sprints, 200 yards each. Walk back to starting point.

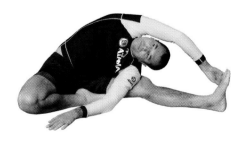

Week 1

Day 3

Warm-Up

PS Static Wall Sit (90): 30 seconds; 30 seconds; 30 seconds

CC Jump Rope (7): 60 seconds; 60 seconds; 60 seconds

Stretch

GSR Gracie Stretch Routine

Strength Training—Plyometrics

PL Medicine Ball Walk (74.1): 15–20 yards; 15–20 yards; 15–20 yards

PL Lateral Jumps—Short Way (70): 20 seconds; 20 seconds; 20 seconds; 20 seconds

PS Power Lunges (85): 15–20 yards; 15–20 yards; 15–20 yards; 15–20 yards

PL Box Jumps—One Leg (67): 8–10; 8–10; 8–10

PL Medicine Ball Toss—Flat Bench (73): 30 seconds; 30 seconds; 30 seconds

PS Ski Jumps (89): 20 seconds; 20 seconds; 20 seconds; 20 seconds

Abdominals

AB Wheels (4): 10–12; 10–12; 10–12; 10–12

AB Medicine Ball Stand-Ups (2): 6–8; 6–8; 6–8; 6–8

Cardiovascular Conditioning

CC Run and Hold (10): 8–10 sets. Run 20 yards and hold for 10 seconds. Your rest period should be 1:20–1:40.

Warm-Up

FW Pullovers—Towel (37): 12; 12; 12

FW Good Mornings (46): 10; 10; 10

Stretch

GSR Gracie Stretch Routine

Strength Training—Chest/Back/Legs

FW Straight-Leg Dead Lifts—Barbell (48): 10; 10; 10

FW Squats—Barbell (44): 10; 10; 8; 8

PL Box Jumps—One Leg (67): 10–14; 10–14; 10–14

ISO Bench Press—Isolateral (57): 10; 8; 6; 6

FW Row—Dumbbell (41): 8; 8; 8; 8

ISO Incline Press—Isolateral (59): 8; 8; 6; 6

FW Towel Pull-Ups (51): 6–8; 6–8; 6–8

Abdominals

AB V-Ups (6): 10–12; 10–12; 10–12; 10–12

Cardiovascular Conditioning

CC Soft Sand Run (11): 20–30 minutes

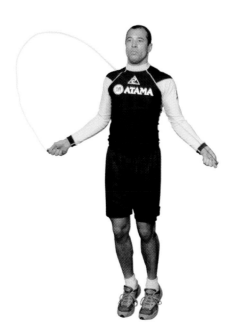

Week 2
Day 1

Warm-Up

FW Rice Grabs (56): 45 seconds; 45 seconds; 45 seconds; 45 seconds

PL Step-Ups—Body Weight (quick feet) (76): 25 seconds; 25 seconds; 25 seconds; 25 seconds

Stretch

GSR Gracie Stretch Routine

Strength Training—Shoulders

ISO Front Raise—Isolateral (58): 10; 10; 10; 10

ISO Lateral Raise—Isolateral (60): 10; 10; 10; 10

FW Shoulder Shrugs—Barbell (42): 10; 10; 10; 10

ISO Military Press—Isolateral (61): 8; 6; 6; 6

FW High Pull—Dumbbell (22): 6; 6; 6; 6

FW Hang Snatch—Dumbbell (23): 5; 5; 5; 5

Abdominals

AB Roll-Ups—Abdominal (3): 15–20; 15–20; 15–20; 15–20

AB V-Ups (6): 10–12; 10–12; 10–12

Cardiovascular Conditioning

CC Steady Run or Jog (12): 5–8 minutes

CC Sprints (13): 4–6 sprints, 200 yards each. Walk back to starting point.

Week 2
Day 2

Warm-Up

PL Medicine Ball Walk (74.1): 20 yards; 20 yards; 20 yards

FW Lunges—Dumbbell (31): 20 reps per side; 20 reps per side; 20 reps per side

CC Jump Rope (7): 60 seconds; 60 seconds; 60 seconds

Stretch

GSR Gracie Stretch Routine

Strength Training—Chest/Back/Legs

PS Squats—Medicine Ball or Plate (91): 15; 15; 15; 15

FW Squats—Barbell (44): 8; 8; 8; 8

PL Box Jumps (use higher box) (66): 8–10; 8–10; 8–10

FW Bench Press—Dumbbell (15): 8; 8; 6; 6; 6

FW Pullovers—Dumbbell (36): 8; 8; 8; 8

ISO Incline Press—Isolateral (59): 8; 8; 8; 8

FW Towel Pull-Ups (51): 6–8; 6–8; 6–8

Abdominals

AB Bench Crunches (1): 20; 20; 20; 20

Cardiovascular Conditioning

CC Steady Run or Jog (12): 5–8 minutes

CC Sprints (13): 4–6 sprints, 200 yards each.
Walk back to starting point.

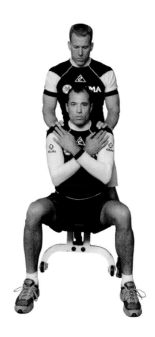

Week 2

Day 3

Warm-Up

PS Static Wall Sit (90): 30 seconds; 30 seconds; 30 seconds

CC Jump Rope (7): 60 seconds; 60 seconds; 60 seconds

Stretch

GSR Gracie Stretch Routine

Strength Training—Plyometrics

PL Medicine Ball Walk (74.1): 15–20 yards; 15–20 yards; 15–20 yards

PL Lateral Jumps—Short Way (70): 20 seconds; 20 seconds; 20 seconds; 20 seconds

PS Power Lunges (85): 15–20 yards; 15–20 yards; 15–20 yards; 15–20 yards

PL Box Jumps (use big box) (66): 8–10; 8–10; 8–10

PL Medicine Ball Toss—Flat Bench (73): 30 seconds; 30 seconds; 30 seconds; 30 seconds

PS Ski Jumps (89): 20 seconds; 20 seconds; 20 seconds; 20 seconds

Abdominals

AB Wheels (4): 10–12; 10–12; 10–12; 10–12

AB Medicine Ball Stand-Ups (2): 6–8; 6–8; 6–8; 6–8

Cardiovascular Conditioning

CC Run and Hold (10): 8–10 sets. Run 20 yards and hold for 10 seconds. Your rest period should be 1:20–1:40.

Week 2
Day 4

Warm-Up

AB V-Ups **(6)**: 10–12; 10–12; 10–12

FW Roll-Ups—Wrist **(40)**: 6–8; 6–8; 6–8

Stretch

GSR Gracie Stretch Routine

Strength Training—Shoulders

ISO Front Raise—Isolateral **(58)**:10; 10; 10; 10

ISO Lateral Raise—Isolateral **(60)**: 10; 10; 10; 10

FW High Pull—Dumbbell **(22)**: 6; 6; 6; 6

FW Hang Snatch—Dumbbell **(23)**: 5; 5; 5; 5

FW Shoulder Shrugs—Barbell **(42)**: 10; 10; 10; 10

ISO Military Press—Isolateral **(61)**: 8; 6; 6; 6

Abdominals

AB Roll-Ups—Abdominal **(3)**: 15–20; 15–20; 15–20; 15–20

Cardiovascular Conditioning

CC Soft Sand Run **(11)**: 20–30 minutes

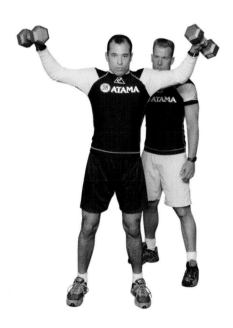

Week 3

Day 1

Warm-Up

FW Reverse Hypers (47): 10; 10; 10

FW Good Mornings (46): 10; 10; 10

CC Jump Rope (7): 60 seconds; 60 seconds; 60 seconds

Stretch

GSR Gracie Stretch Routine

Strength Training—Chest/Back/Legs

PS Step-Ups—Barbell (92): 8 per leg; 8 per leg; 8 per leg; 8 per leg

PS Squats—Medicine Ball or Plate (91): 15; 15; 15

FW Squats—Barbell (44): 8; 8; 6; 6

FW Pullovers—Barbell (35): 8; 8; 6; 6

FW Bench Press—Barbell (14): 10; 8; 8; 6; 6

FW Row—Dumbbell (41): 8; 8; 6; 6

FW Incline Press—Barbell (24): 8; 8; 6; 6

Abdominals

AB Wheels (4): 12–14; 12–14; 12–14

AB Medicine Ball Stand-Ups (2): 6–8; 6–8; 6–8

Cardiovascular Conditioning

CC Sprints (13): 4 150-yard sprints, 6 100-yard sprints. Walk back to starting point.

CC Steady Run or Jog (12): 5–8 minutes

Week 3
Day 2

Warm-Up

FW Rice Grabs (56): 45 seconds; 45 seconds; 45 seconds

PL Step-Ups—Body Weight (quick feet) (76): 30 seconds; 30 seconds; 30 seconds

Stretch

GSR Gracie Stretch Routine

Strength Training—Shoulders

FW Front Raise—Barbell (17): 10; 10; 10; 10

FW Lateral Raise—Dumbbell (28): 8; 8; 8; 8

FW Push Press—Barbell (38): 8; 8; 6; 6

FW Shoulder Shrugs—Barbell (42): 10; 10; 10; 10

FW Upright Row—Barbell (52): 8; 8; 6; 6

Abdominals

AB V-Ups (6): 15–18; 15–18; 15–18

AB Roll-Ups—Abdominal (3): 20–25; 20–25; 20–25

Cardiovascular Conditioning

CC Soft Sand Run (11) or Steady Run or Jog (12): 25–30 minutes

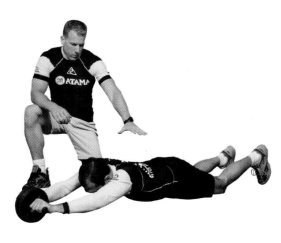

Week 3

Day 3

Warm-Up

PS Static Wall Sit (90): 30 seconds; 30 seconds; 30 seconds

CC Jump rope (7): 60 seconds; 60 seconds; 60 seconds

Stretch

GSR Gracie Stretch Routine

Strength Training—Plyometrics

PS Ski Jumps (89): 30 seconds; 30 seconds; 30 seconds

PS Lateral Shuffle—Double Plate (80): 20 seconds; 20 seconds; 20 seconds

PS Cones Workout (Figure 8s—Standing) (77.1): 20 seconds; 20 seconds; 20 seconds

PL Box Jumps (66): 6–8; 6–8; 6–8

PL Medicine Ball Walk (74.1): 15–20 yards; 15–20 yards; 15–20 yards

PS Knee-Ups (78): 40; 40; 40

Abdominals

AB Bench Crunches (1): 25; 25; 25

FW Good Mornings (46): 15; 15; 15

Cardiovascular Conditioning

CC Sprints (13): 10–12 sprints, 100 yards each. You have 60 seconds to sprint 100 yards and jog back to starting point.

Week 3

Day 4

Warm-Up

FW **Reverse Hypers (47):** 12–15; 12–15; 12–15

FW **Good Mornings (46):** 12–15; 12–15; 12–15

Stretch

GSR Gracie Stretch Routine

Strength Training—Chest/Back/Legs

FW **Lunges—Dumbbell (31):** 20 reps per side; 20 reps per side; 20 reps per side

PL **Push-Ups—Plyometric (75):** 8–10; 8–10; 8–10

FW **Towel Pull-Ups (51):** 8-10; 8-10; 8-10; 8-10

FW **Bench Press—Barbell (14):** 10; 8; 8; 6; 6

FW **Bench Press—Narrow Grip Barbell (16):** 8; 8; 8

FW **Pullovers—Barbell (35):** 8; 8; 8; 8

FW **Incline Press—Barbell (24):** 8; 8; 6; 6

Abdominals

AB **V-Ups (6):** 15–20; 15–20; 15–20; 15–20

Cardiovascular Conditioning

CC **Run and Hold (10):** 10 sets. Run 20 yards and hold for 10 seconds. Your rest period should be 1 minute–1:20.

CC **Steady Run or Jog (12):** 5–8 minutes

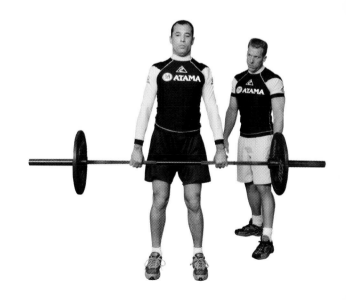

Week 4

Day 1

Warm-Up

FW Roll-Ups—Wrist (40): 6–8; 6–8; 6–8

PS Step-Ups—Body Weight (quick feet) (76): 30 seconds; 30 seconds; 30 seconds

Stretch

GSR Gracie Stretch Routine

Strength Training —Shoulders

FW **ISO** Front Raise—Dumbell (18) *or* Isolateral (58): 8; 8; 8; 8

FW **ISO** Lateral Raise—Dumbbell (28) *or* Isolateral (60): 8; 8; 8; 8

FW Hang Snatch—Dumbbell (23): 5; 5; 4; 4

FW High Pull—Dumbbell (22): 5; 5; 4; 4

FW Military Press—Narrow Grip Barbell (34): 8; 8; 6; 6

FW Upright Row—Dumbbell (53): 8; 8; 6; 6

Abdominals

AB Wheels (4): 12–14; 12–14; 12–14

FW Good Mornings (46): 15; 15; 15

Cardiovascular Conditioning

CC Sprints (13): 4 150-yard sprints, 6 100-yard sprints. Walk back to starting point.

CC Steady Run or Jog (12): 5–8 minutes

Week 4
Day 2

Warm-Up

PL Medicine Ball Walk (74.1): 20 yards; 20 yards; 20 yards

PS Power Lunges (85): 20 yards; 20 yards; 20 yards

Stretch

GSR Gracie Stretch Routine

Strength Training—Chest/Back/Legs

PS Squats—Medicine Ball or Plate (91): 15; 15; 15

FW Squats—Barbell (44): 8; 8; 6; 6

FW Bench Press—Barbell (14): 10; 8; 8; 6; 6

FW Row—Dumbbell (20): 8; 8; 6; 6

FW Incline Press—Barbell (24): 8; 8; 6; 6

FW Towel Pull-Ups (51): 6–8; 6–8; 6–8

PS Medicine Ball Toss—Chest (83): 8–10; 8–10; 8–10

Abdominals

AB Wheels (4): 12–14; 12–14; 12–14

AB Medicine Ball Stand-Ups (2): 6–8; 6–8; 6–8

Cardiovascular Conditioning

CC Steady Run or Jog (12): 25–30 minutes

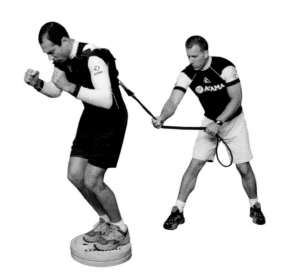

Week 4

Day 3

Warm-Up

PS Medicine Ball Toss—Overhead (84): 8–10; 8–10; 8–10

PS Static Wall Sit (90): 30 seconds; 30 seconds; 30 seconds

Stretch

GSR Gracie Stretch Routine

Strength Training—Plyometrics

PL Lateral Jumps—Long Way (69): 20 seconds; 20 seconds; 20 seconds

PS Power Lunges (85): 15–20 yards; 15–20 yards; 15–20 yards; 15–20 yards

PS Cones Workout (Figure 8s—Standing) (77.1): 30 seconds; 30 seconds; 30 seconds; 30 seconds

PL Box Jumps (quick feet) (66): 20; 20; 20; 20

PS Knee-Ups (78): 40; 40; 40; 40

PS Ski Jumps (89): 30 seconds; 30 seconds; 30 seconds

Abdominals

AB Bench Crunches (1): 25; 25; 25; 25

FW Good Mornings (46): 15; 15; 15; 15

Cardiovascular Conditioning

CC Sprints (13): 10–12 sprints, 100 yards each. You have 60 seconds to sprint 100 yards and jog back to starting point.

Week 4
Day 4

Warm-Up

FW Reverse Hypers (47): 12–15; 12–15; 12–15

FW Rice Grabs (56): 45 seconds; 45 seconds; 45 seconds

Stretch

GSR Gracie Stretch Routine

Strength Training—Legs and Shoulders

FW Straight-Leg Dead Lifts—Dumbbell (49): 10; 10; 10; 10

FW Squats—Dumbbell (45): 10; 10; 8; 8

FW Shoulder Shrugs—Dumbbell (43): 10; 10; 10; 10

FW Lateral Raise—Dumbbell (28): 8; 8; 8; 8

FW Push Press—Dumbbell (39): 8; 8; 6; 6

FW Hang Clean—Dumbbell (21): 5; 5; 4; 4

FW Upright Row—Barbell (52): 8; 8; 6; 6

Abdominals

AB V-Ups (6): 15–20; 15–20; 15–20; 15–20

Cardiovascular Conditioning

CC Run and Hold (10): 10 sets. Run 20 yards and hold for 10 seconds. Your rest period should be 1 minute–1:20

CC Steady Run or Jog (12): 5–8 minutes

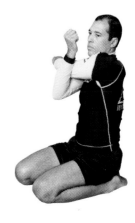

ADVANCED WORKOUT AW

5 days/week

The advanced workout should be six weeks long. Start the workout with the two-week routine described below, then go back to the intermediate workout, using the routine described there but adding an exercise to each day from the strength training group of that day. For example, if the strength training is focused on plyometrics that day, add another plyometric exercise; if it is focused on legs, add a leg exercise. Use the number of reps and sets that is given for the exercise (or for similar exercises) elsewhere in the intermediate routine.

Week 1
Day 1

Warm-Up

AB V-Ups (6): 10–12; 10–12; 10–12

FW Roll-Ups—Wrist (40): 6–8; 6–8; 6–8

Stretch

GSR Gracie Stretch Routine

Strength Training—Shoulders

ISO Lateral Raise—Isolateral (60): 10; 10; 10; 10

FW Front Raise—Dumbbell (18): 10; 10; 10; 10

FW High Pull—Dumbbell (22): 6; 6; 6; 6

FW Hang Snatch—Dumbbell (23): 5; 5; 5; 5

FW Shoulder Shrugs—Barbell (42): 10; 10; 10; 10

FW Military Press—Dumbbell (33): 8; 6; 6; 6

Abdominals

AB Roll-Ups—Abdominal (3): 15–20; 15–20; 15–20; 15–20

Cardiovascular Conditioning

CC Soft Sand Run (11): 20–30 minutes

Warm-Up

FW **Reverse Hypers (47):** 10; 10; 10

FW **Good Mornings (46):** 10; 10; 10

CC **Jump Rope (7):** 60 seconds; 60 seconds; 60 seconds

Stretch

GSR **Gracie Stretch Routine**

Strength Training—Legs/Chest/Back

PS **Step-Ups—Barbell (92):** 8 per leg; 8 per leg; 8 per leg; 8 per leg

PS **Squats—Medicine Ball or Plate (91):** 15; 15; 15

FW **Squats—Barbell (44):** 8; 8; 6; 6

FW **Pullovers—Barbell (35):** 8; 8; 6; 6

FW **Bench Press—Barbell (14):** 10; 8; 8; 6; 6

FW **Row—Dumbbell (41):** 8; 8; 6; 6

FW **Incline Press—Barbell (24):** 8; 8; 6; 6

Abdominals

AB **Wheels (4):** 12–14; 12–14; 12–14

AB **Medicine Ball Stand-Ups (2):** 6–8; 6–8; 6–8

Cardiovascular Conditioning

CC **Sprints (13):** 4 150-yard sprints, 6 100-yard sprints. Walk back to starting point.

CC **Steady Run or Jog (12):** 5–8 minutes

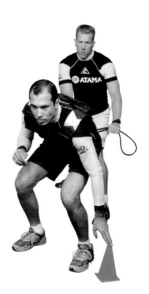

Week 1

Day 3

Warm-Up

FW Rice Grabs (56): 45 seconds; 45 seconds; 45 seconds

PL Step-Ups—Body Weight (quick feet) (76): 30 seconds; 30 seconds; 30 seconds

Stretch

GSR Gracie Stretch Routine

Strength Training—Shoulders

FW Front Raise—Barbell (17): 10; 10; 10; 10

FW Lateral Raise—Dumbbell (28): 8; 8; 8; 8

FW Push Press—Barbell (38): 8; 8; 6; 6

FW Shoulder Shrugs—Barbell (42): 10; 10; 10; 10

FW Upright Row—Barbell (52): 8; 8; 6; 6

Abdominals

AB V-Ups (6): 15–18; 15–18; 15–18

AB Roll-Ups—Abdominal (3): 20–25; 20–25; 20–25

Cardiovascular Conditioning

CC Soft Sand Run (11): 25–30 minutes

Week 1
Day 4

Warm-Up

PS Static Wall Sit (90): 30 seconds; 30 seconds; 30 seconds

CC Jump Rope (7): 60 seconds; 60 seconds; 60 seconds

Stretch

GSR Gracie Stretch Routine

Strength Training—Plyometrics

PS Ski Jumps (89): 30 seconds; 30 seconds; 30 seconds

PS Lateral Shuffle—Double Plate (80): 30 seconds; 30 seconds; 30 seconds

PS Cones Workout (Figure 8s—Push-Ups) (77.2): 30 seconds; 30 seconds; 30 seconds

PL Box Jumps (use big box) (66): 6–8; 6–8; 6–8

PL Medicine Ball Walk (74.1): 15–20 yards; 15–20 yards; 15–20 yards

PS Knee-Ups (78): 40; 40; 40

Abdominals

AB Bench Crunches (1): 25; 25; 25

FW Good Mornings (46): 15; 15; 15

Cardiovascular Conditioning

CC Sprints (13): 10–12 sprints, 100 yards each. You have 60 seconds to sprint 100 yards and jog back to starting point.

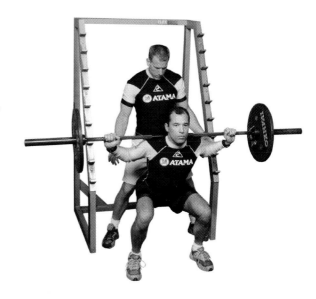

Week 1

Day 5

Warm-Up

FW **Reverse Hypers (47):** 12–15; 12–15; 12–15

FW **Good Mornings (46):** 12–15; 12–15; 12–15

Stretch

GSR Gracie Stretch Routine

Strength Training—Legs/Chest/Back

FW **Lunges—Dumbbell (31):** 20 reps per side; 20 reps per side; 20 reps per side; 20 reps per side

PL **Push-Ups—Plyometric (75):** 8–10; 8–10; 8–10; 8–10

FW **Towel Pulls–Ups (51):** 8–10; 8–10; 8–10; 8–10

FW **Bench Press—Barbell (14):** 10; 8; 8; 6; 6

FW **Bench Press—Narrow Grip Barbell (16):** 8; 8; 8

FW **Pullovers—Barbell (35):** 8; 8; 8; 8

FW **Incline Press—Barbell (24):** 8; 8; 6; 6

Abdominals

AB **V-Ups (6):** 15–20; 15–20; 15–20; 15–20

Cardiovascular Conditioning

CC **Run and Hold (10):** 10 sets. Run 20 yards and hold for 10 seconds. Your rest period should be 1 minute–1:20

CC **Steady Run or Jog (12):** 5–8 minutes

Week 2
Day 1

Warm-Up

FW Roll-Ups—Wrist (40): 6–8; 6–8; 6–8

PL Step-Ups—Body Weight (quick feet) (76): 30 seconds; 30 seconds; 30 seconds

Stretch

GSR Gracie Stretch Routine

Strength Training—Shoulders

ISO Front Raise—Isolateral (58): 8; 8; 8; 8

FW Lateral Raise—Dumbbell (28): 8; 8; 8; 8

FW Hang Snatch—Dumbbell (23): 5; 5; 4; 4

FW High Pull—Dumbbell (22): 5; 5; 4; 4

FW Military Press—Narrow Grip Barbell (34): 8; 8; 6; 6

FW Upright Row—Dumbbell (53): 8; 8; 6; 6

Abdominals

AB Wheels (4): 12–14; 12–14; 12–14

Cardiovascular Conditioning

CC Sprints (13): 4 150-yard sprints, 6 100-yard sprints. Walk back to starting point.

CC Steady Run or Jog (12): 5–8 minutes

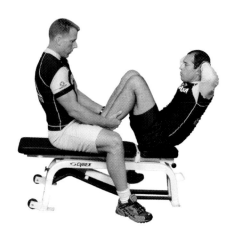

Week 2

Day 2

Warm-Up

PL Medicine Ball Walk (74.1): 20 yards; 20 yards; 20 yards

PS Power Lunges (85): 20 yards; 20 yards; 20 yards

Stretch

GSR Gracie Stretch Routine

Strength Training—Legs/Chest/Back

PS Squats—Medicine Ball or Plate (91): 15; 15; 15

FW Squats—Dumbbell (45): 8; 8; 6; 6

FW Bench Press—Barbell (14): 10; 8; 8; 6; 6

FW Row—Dumbbell (41): 8; 8; 6; 6

FW Incline Press—Barbell (24): 8; 8; 6; 6

FW Towel Pull–Ups (51): 6–8; 6–8; 6–8

PS Medicine Ball Toss—Chest (83): 8–10; 8–10; 8–10

Abdominals

AB Wheels (4): 12–14; 12–14; 12–14

AB Medicine Ball Stand-Ups (2): 6–8; 6–8; 6–8

Cardiovascular Conditioning

CC Soft Sand Run (11): 25–30 minutes

Week 2
Day 3

Warm-Up

PS Medicine Ball Toss—Overhead (84): 8–10; 8–10; 8–10

PS Static Wall Sit (90): 30 seconds; 30 seconds; 30 seconds

Stretch

GSR Gracie Stretch Routine

Strength Training—Plyometrics

PL Lateral Jumps—Long Way (69): 30 seconds; 30 seconds; 30 seconds

PS Power Lunges (85): 15–20 yards; 15–20 yards; 15–20 yards; 15–20 yards

PS Cones Workout (Figure 8s—Push-Ups) (77.2): 30 seconds; 30 seconds; 30 seconds; 30 seconds

PL Box Jumps (quick feet) (66): 20; 20; 20; 20

PS Knee-Ups (78): 40; 40; 40; 40

PS Ski Jumps (89): 30 seconds; 30 seconds; 30 seconds

Abdominals

AB Bench Crunches (1): 25; 25; 25; 25

FW Good Mornings (46): 15; 15; 15; 15

Cardiovascular Conditioning

CC Sprints (13): 10–12 sprints, 100 yards each. You have 60 seconds to sprint 100 yards and jog back to starting point.

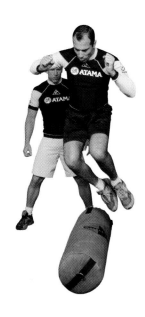

Week 2

Day 4

Warm-Up

FW **Reverse Hypers (47):** 12–15; 12–15; 12–15

FW **Rice Grabs (56):** 45 seconds; 45 seconds; 45 seconds

Stretch

GSR Gracie Stretch Routine

Strength Training—Legs and Shoulders

FW **Straight-Leg Dead Lifts—Barbell (48):** 10; 10; 10; 10

FW **Squats—Dumbbell (45):** 10; 10; 8; 8

FW **Shoulder Shrugs—Dumbbell (Hands-on) (43a):** 10; 10; 10; 10

FW **Lateral Raise—Dumbbell Seated (29):** 8; 8; 8; 8

FW **Push Press—Dumbbell (39):** 8; 8; 6; 6

FW **Hang Clean—Dumbbell (21):** 5; 5; 4; 4

FW **Upright Row—Barbell (52):** 8; 8; 6; 6

Abdominals

AB **V-Ups (6):** 15–20; 15–20; 15–20; 15–20

Cardiovascular Conditioning

CC **Run and Hold (10):** 10 sets. Run 20 yards and hold for 10 seconds. Your rest period should be 1 minute–1:20.

CC **Steady Run or Jog (12):** 5–8 minutes

Warm-Up

PS Static Wall Sit (90): 30 seconds; 30 seconds; 30 seconds

CC Jump Rope (7): 60 seconds; 60 seconds; 60 seconds

Stretch

GSR Gracie Stretch Routine

Strength Training—Plyometrics

PS Ski Jumps (89): 30 seconds; 30 seconds; 30 seconds

PS Lateral Shuffle—Double Plate (80): 30 seconds; 30 seconds; 30 seconds

PS Cones Workout (Figure 8s—Push-Ups) (77.2): 30 seconds; 30 seconds; 30 seconds

PL Box Jumps (use big box) (66): 6–8; 6–8; 6–8

PL Medicine Ball Walk (74.1): 15–20 yards; 15–20 yards; 15–20 yards

PS Knee-Ups (78): 40; 40; 40

Abdominals

AB Bench Crunches (1): 25; 25; 25

FW Good Mornings (46): 15; 15; 15

Cardiovascular Conditioning

CC Sprints (13): 10–12 sprints, 100 yards each. You have 60 seconds to sprint 100 yards and jog back to starting point.

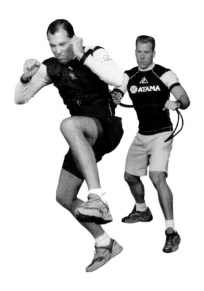

— PART FOUR —

Royce's Family Diet

You've heard it a million times, but it couldn't be more true: You are what you eat! Every cell of your body is built from the food you consume. There is no way to have a healthy body unless you feed it healthy food.

Now, having said that, we think you should throw out whatever diet advice you've been following. People go crazy trying to follow very specific diets, when the fact of the matter is that they don't have to in order to stay healthy. If you are a martial artist, you are getting plenty of exercise and burning lots of calories each day, so all you really need to do is make sure you feed your body plenty of protein (meat, fish, beans, nuts, and tofu) for muscle building, and quality carbohydrates (starches and fruits) for energy. Mix in some healthy fats (olive or canola oil), some veggies, and some calcium for building bone, and you're good to go.

That much nutritional info you could get anywhere, but we're going to let you in on our secret now: Lots of athletes eat a healthy mix of proteins, carbs, and veggies and still never feel as good as they could and never excel in competition. The reason is that they combine the wrong foods at the wrong times, and even though the foods are all healthy, they cancel out each other's beneficial effects. This is the core of Royce's Family Diet: learning about how foods work together to keep you healthy.

Royce's family diet was developed in Brazil by his uncle Carlos. As he became older, Carlos grew very interested in the ways that foods worked in combination. He researched the healing methods of indigenous cultures in Brazil's Amazon rainforest and applied those teachings to modern diets. He also spent decades of trial and error learning what worked and what didn't. The result is a unique system of dietary wisdom that almost all the Gracies follow. They hold the diet responsible for the high level of functioning—and rarity of illness—they have maintained over the years.

Here is how Royce explains it:

The diet is for easy digestion. I can't get to a fight and be feeling bad because of the meal that I ate. I can't afford to miss a week of training because I'm sick. I can't abandon a seminar because I don't feel up to teaching. If you have heartburn or indigestion, that means your body is not concentrating on improving, staying healthy, or healing an injury. Your body is fighting the meal rather than getting benefits from it.

During training for a specific fight, I will supplement the diet. I normally have three meals a day, but when I am training I do add protein shakes and protein bars. So if I am not in training, I have three meals a day. When I gear up for a fight, I add three protein shakes a day, so I have six meals a day: three meals consisting of food and three others of protein shakes. I may also add protein bars to the regular food meals, so the body can have enough fuel to sustain the extra effort that I am demanding of it.

The last few days prior to the fight, I will eat more pasta. Especially the day before the fight, I add the carbohydrates. That way my body will have plenty of carbs to burn and won't have to try to get its fuel from protein, which would decrease my power. It is the same principle as the marathon runners use: the last two days prior to the fight I load up with carbs.

Royce's Family Diet isn't hard to follow once you know a few basic rules. The trick is learning which foods fall into which groups, and then learning the rules about combining groups. But remember, as with the rest of any fitness system, don't expect immediate results. The benefits are gradual. Much in the same way as you don't drop dead on the spot when you eat something that is bad for you, or do something unhealthy like smoking, the benefits of a new lifestyle and new diet are slow to come but will greatly add to your ability to perform and feel good. After a while, you will have greater energy and vitality. You will sleep better and your body will be able to heal faster and recuperate faster, as well. When you eat right, you give your body the raw material that it needs to perform at its peak!

Food Groups

Group A: Proteins, vegetables, and fats (meat, fish, vegetables, nuts, and oils)

Group B: Carbohydrates (grains, pasta, beans, bread, rice)

Group C: Sweet fruits, fresh cheeses (such as cream cheese), and sugar and other sweeteners

Group D: Acidic fruits (citrus, berries, etc.) and sour dairy products (yogurt, buttermilk)

Group E: Sweet dairy products

Rules

- Foods from Group A combine with each other plus ONE from group B.
- Foods from Group C combine with each other plus ONE from group B.
- Foods from Group B do not combine with each other but combine with Groups A or C.
- Foods from Group D do not combine with each other or any other group. They must be eaten alone.
- Foods from Group E combine with all of Group B and C but none of Group A.

No-Nos

- No snacking. Wait five hours between meals for full digestion.
- No alcohol. Drink lots of water instead.
- No dessert. It impedes the absorption of your dinner nutrients.
- No aged cheeses or vinegar. Aged cheeses have a high fat content. Vinegar is pure acid, which cannot mix with anything else—and you can't eat a meal of vinegar alone.
- No processed foods, or as few as possible.

Following these rules can take some getting used to for those accustomed to the typical American diet. For example, the common habit of drinking orange juice with breakfast does not work with the Gracie Diet because oranges are acidic (Group C) and do not mix with any other food type. You must change your morning juice to apple, guava, or something else less acidic.

Another rule that throws a lot of people is the starch rule. Starches don't combine with each other, so if you have a hamburger with a bun (wheat), you can't eat french fries (potato) at the same time. In this case, do what Royce does: ditch the bun and eat the fries. Make up the lack of one by increased quantities. For instance, when Royce has a morning meal of oranges, he will eat three dozen oranges! He may either juice them or simply chew on them to get the juice and spit the pulp. When he goes out for a burger and fries, he may eat two or three burger patties and a basket of fries! The important thing is to eat enough to satisfy your nutritional needs, but stay within the food combinations!

When he is preparing for fights, Royce supplements his diet with protein bars and shakes. He prefers protein bars from PowerBar—peanut butter and vanilla—and shakes from Met-Max and Pro-Score, which he mixes with Power Glutamine from Champion Nutrition and drinks at night. For recovery during the day, he drinks Champion Nutrition's Revenge, which is similar to Gatorade. He also relies on acai, a berry from the Brazilian rainforest that the Gracies have been using for generations to supercharge their performance. Amazonian tribal warriors consumed acai mixed with guaraná for centuries to increase strength, heighten awareness, and improve mental clarity. Today, scientific studies have revealed that acai is rich in antioxidants and omega 3, 6, and 9 fatty acids. The Health Science Institute named it a superfood, and Royce uses it all the time! Acai can be purchased online from www.sambazon.com or www.zolaacai.com and many retail stores stock it on their shelves.

The following is Royce's own informal meal plan for one month. The first 19 days represent meals he would eat while training at home, and the next 12 are for time spent on the road during seminars. By seeing both types of meal plans, you can learn to eat within the diet even when you have to have meals out of town or at work, when you may have to have fast food!

Training at Home

Day 1

BK Cheese omelet with hash browns
LU Tuna sandwich
DN Pasta salad with salmon

Day 2

BK Orange juice
LU Veggie lasagna, salad, shrimp, asparagus, and cashews
DN Apple juice, toast, cheese, and honey

Day 3

BK Banana and milk
LU Veggie lasagna, salad, and shrimp
DN Pear juice, banana, bread with cheese

Day 4

BK Strawberry juice
LU Salad, beef stroganoff, rice, and carrot juice
DN Guava juice and blueberry muffin

Day 5

BK Banana and milk
LU Turkey sandwich, salad, and fried zucchini
DN Beef stroganoff with bread and carrot juice

Day 6

BK Protein shake
LU Chicken romano and pasta
DN Papaya, apple juice, cream cheese, and honey (all blended)

Day 7

BK Banana and milk
LU Mushroom burger—no bun—and French fries
DN Papaya, cream cheese, and honey

Day 8

BK Acai and a cheese sandwich
LU Tuna melt
DN Grilled mahi-mahi, baked potato, and salad

Day 9

BK Cheese omelet and hash browns
LU Skip
DN Grilled swordfish salad, calamari, and baked potato

Day 10

BK Yogurt
LU turkey sandwich and salad
DN Watermelon juice and cheese sandwich

Day 11

BK Orange juice
LU Chicken and veggie omelet with avocado and toast
DN Apple juice and cheese sandwich

Day 12

BK Acai and banana
LU Turkey sandwich with avocado and lettuce
DN Banana muffin, gouda cheese, and guava juice

Day 13

BK Banana and milk
LU Mushroom and green pepper omelet (egg whites only) with croissant
DN Caesar salad, fresh mozzarella, angel hair pasta with chicken

Day 14

BK Acai, banana, cream cheese, and crushed ice smoothie
LU Grilled fish, rice, and cashews
DN Watermelon juice, banana muffin, and cheese

Day 15

BK None
LU Steak wrap
DN Baked halibut with mushrooms, bell pepper, and a melted cheese sandwich

Day 16

BK Cheese omelet (egg whites only) with hash browns
LU Chicken and black beans
DN Watermelon juice, cheese, dates, wheat bread

Day 17

BK Acai, cream cheese, banana, and crushed ice smoothie
LU Turkey sandwich with lettuce and mayo
DN Chicken pizza with cashews, avocado, and carrot juice

Day 18

BK Protein shake
LU Tuna melt
DN Guava juice, jack cheese sandwich, and dates